Tactical Combat Casualty Care
and
Wound Treatment

U.S. Department of Defense

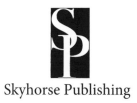

Skyhorse Publishing

Skyhorse Publishing books may be purchased in bulk at special discounts for sales promotion, corporate gifts, fund-raising, or educational purposes. Special editions can also be created to specifications. For details, contact the Special Sales Department, Skyhorse Publishing, 307 West 36th Street, 11th Floor, New York, NY 10018 or info@skyhorsepublishing.com.

Skyhorse® and Skyhorse Publishing® are registered trademarks of Skyhorse Publishing, Inc.®, a Delaware corporation.

Visit our website at www.skyhorsepublishing.com.

10 9 8 7 6 5 4

Library of Congress Cataloging-in-Publication Data is available on file.

Cover design by Brian Peterson

ISBN: 978-1-63450-331-0
Ebook ISBN: 978-1-63450-960-2

Printed in China

DEVELOPMENT

This subcourse is approved for resident and correspondence course instruction. It reflects the current thought of the Academy of Health Sciences and conforms to printed Department of the Army doctrine as closely as currently possible. Development and progress render such doctrine continuously subject to change.

ADMINISTRATION

Students who desire credit hours for this correspondence subcourse must enroll in the subcourse. Application for enrollment should be made at the Internet website: http://www.atrrs.army.mil. You can access the course catalog in the upper right corner. Enter School Code 555 for medical correspondence courses. Copy down the course number and title. To apply for enrollment, return to the main ATRRS screen and scroll down the right side for ATRRS Channels. Click on SELF DEVELOPMENT to open the application; then follow the on-screen instructions.

For comments or questions regarding enrollment, student records, or examination shipments, contact the Nonresident Instruction Branch at DSN 471-5877, commercial (210) 221-5877, toll-free 1-800-344-2380; fax: 210-221-4012 or DSN 471-4012, email accp@amedd.army.mil, or write to:

NONRESIDENT INSTRUCTION BRANCH
AMEDDC&S
ATTN: MCCS-HSN
2105 11TH STREET SUITE 4191
FORT SAM HOUSTON TX 78234-5064

Be sure your social security number is on all correspondence sent to the Academy of Health Sciences.

CLARIFICATION OF TERMINOLOGY

When used in this publication, words such as "he," "him," "his," and "men" 'are intended to include both the masculine and feminine genders, unless specifically stated otherwise or when obvious in context.

USE OF PROPRIETARY NAMES

The initial letters of the names of some products may be capitalized in this subcourse. Such names are proprietary names, that is, brand names or trademarks. Proprietary names have been used in this subcourse only to make it a more effective learning aid. The use of any name, proprietary or otherwise, should not be interpreted as endorsement, deprecation, or criticism of a product; nor should such use be considered to interpret the validity of proprietary rights in a name, whether it is registered or not.

TABLE OF CONTENTS

SUBCOURSE MD0554

TACTICAL COMBAT CASUALTY CARE AND WOUND TREATMENT

INTRODUCTION

When you have casualties on the battlefield, you must determine the sequence in which the casualties are to be treated and how to treat their injuries. This subcourse discusses the procedures for performing tactical combat casualty care; treating injuries to the extremities, chest, abdominal, and head; and controlling shock.

Subcourse Components:

This subcourse consists of eight lessons. The lessons are:

Lesson 1, Tactical Combat Casualty Care.

Lesson 2, Controlling Bleeding From an Extremity.

Lesson 3, Treating Chest Injuries.

Lesson 4, Treating Abdominal Injuries.

Lesson 5, Treating Head Injuries.

Lesson 6, Treating Burns.

Lesson 7, Treating Hypovolemic Shock.

Lesson 8, Treating Soft Tissue Injuries.

Here are some suggestions that may be helpful to you in completing this subcourse:

--Read and study each lesson carefully.

--Complete the subcourse lesson by lesson. After completing each lesson, work the exercises at the end of the lesson, marking your answers in this booklet.

--After completing each set of lesson exercises, compare your answers with those on the solution sheet that follows the exercises. If you have answered an exercise incorrectly, check the reference cited after the answer on the solution sheet to determine why your response was not the correct one.

Credit Awarded:

Upon successful completion of the examination for this subcourse, you will be awarded 16 credit hours.

To receive credit hours, you must be officially enrolled and complete an examination furnished by the Nonresident Instruction Section at Fort Sam Houston, Texas.

You can enroll by going to the web site http://atrrs.army.mil and enrolling under "Self Development" (School Code 555).

A listing of correspondence courses and subcourses available through the Nonresident Instruction Section is found in Chapter 4 of DA Pamphlet 350-59, Army Correspondence Course Program Catalog. The DA PAM is available at the following website: http://www.usapa.army.mil/pdffiles/p350-59.pdf.

LESSON ASSIGNMENT

LESSON 1	Tactical Combat Casualty Care.
TEXT ASSIGNMENT	Paragraphs 1-1 through 1-5.
LESSON OBJECTIVES	When you have completed this lesson, you should be able to:

    1-1. Identify factors that influence combat casualty care.

    1-2. Identify the stages of care?

    1-3. Identify the procedures for care under fire.

    1-4. Identify the procedures for tactical field care.

    1-5. Identify the procedures for casualty evacuation care.

SUGGESTION   Work the lesson exercises at the end of this lesson before beginning the next lesson. These exercises will help you accomplish the lesson objectives.

LESSON 1

TACTICAL COMBAT CASUALTY CARE

1-1. GENERAL

As a combat medic on today's battlefield, you will experience a wide variety of conditions not previously experienced. Your training has prepared you on standards that apply to the civilian emergency medical service (EMS) world that may not apply to the combat environment. These tools are a good basis for sound medical judgment; on today's battlefield, this judgment could save the lives of your fellow soldiers. The US Army found the need to migrate away from the civilian standards and allow the combat medics to analyze situations in ways not previously thought of. These techniques are called "tactical combat casualty care" (TC3). These techniques and factors will be discussed in the following paragraphs. Factors influencing combat casualty care include the following.

a. **Enemy Fire**. It may prevent the treatment of casualties and may put you at risk in providing care under enemy fire.

b. **Medical Equipment Limitations**. You only have what you carried in with you in your medical aid bag.

c. **A Widely Variable Evacuation Time**. In the civilian community, evacuation can be under 25 minutes; but in combat, evacuation may be delayed for several hours.

d. **Tactical Considerations**. Sometimes the mission will take precedence over medical care.

e. **Casualty Transportation**. Transportation for evacuation may or may not be available. Air superiority must be achieved before any air evacuation assets will be deployed. Additionally, the tactical situation will dictate when or if casualty evacuation can occur. In addition, environmental factors may prevent evacuation assets from reaching your casualty.

1-2. STAGES OF CARE

In making the transition from civilian emergency care to the tactical setting, it is useful in considering the management of casualties that occurs in a combat mission as being divided into three distinct phases.

a. **Care Under Fire**. Care under fire is the care rendered by the soldier medic at the scene of the injury while he and the casualty are still under effective hostile fire. Available medical equipment is limited to that carried by the individual soldier or the soldier medic in his medical aid bag.

b. **Tactical Field Care**. Tactical field care is the care rendered by the soldier medic once he and the casualty are no longer under effective hostile fire. It also applies to situations in which an injury has occurred, but there is no hostile fire. Available medical equipment is still limited to that being carried into the field by medical personnel. The time needed to evacuate the casualty to a medical treatment facility (MTF) may vary considerably.

c. **Combat Casualty Evacuation Care**. Combat casualty evacuation (CASEVAC) care is the care rendered once the casualty has been picked up by an aircraft, vehicle, or boat. Additional medical personnel and equipment may have been pre-staged and are available at this stage of casualty management.

1-3. CARE UNDER FIRE

a. Medical personnel's firepower may be essential in obtaining tactical fire superiority. Attention to suppression of hostile fire may minimize the risk of injury to personnel and minimize additional injury to previously injured soldiers. The best offense on the battlefield is tactical fire superiority. There is little time available to provide care while under enemy fire and it may be more important to suppress enemy fire than stopping to care for casualties. The tactical situation will dictate when and how much care you can provide. Finally, when a medical evacuation (MEDEVAC) is requested, the tactical situation may not safely allow the air asset to respond.

b. Personnel may need to assist in returning fire instead of stopping to care for casualties. This may include wounded soldiers that are still able to fight.

c. Wounded soldiers who are unable to fight and who are exposed to enemy fire should move as quickly as possible to any nearby cover. If no cover is available or the wounded soldier cannot move to cover, he should lie flat and motionless (play dead).

d. Figure 1-1 depicts a tragic situation. A wounded Marine is down in the street. A colleague attempts to come to his rescue along with a second Marine. Enemy fire continues in the area and the first rescuer is critically wounded. The second rescuer returns behind cover. Eventually, after enemy fire is contained, the first wounded Marine is rescued and the initial rescuer is permanently disabled. The point is, when under enemy fire, we cannot afford to rush blindly into a danger area to rescue a fallen comrade. If we do, there may be additional soldiers wounded or killed attempting to rescue our wounded.

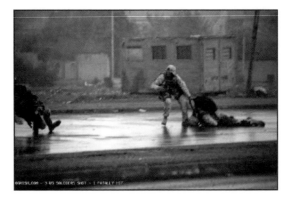

Figure 1-1. Soldier and rescuers wounded.

    e. Medical personnel are limited and, if they are injured, no other medical personnel will be available until the time of evacuation during the CASEVAC phase.

    f.   No immediate management of the airway is necessary at this time due to the limited time available while under enemy fire and during the movement of the casualty to cover. Airway problems typically play a minimal role in combat casualties. Wounding data from Viet Nam indicates airway problems were present in only about one percent of combat casualties, mostly from maxillofacial injuries.

    g. The control of hemorrhage (major bleeding) is important since injury to a major vessel can result in hypovolemic shock in a short time frame. Extremity hemorrhage is the leading cause of preventable combat death.

NOTE: Over 2,500 deaths occurred in Viet Nam secondary to hemorrhage from extremity wounds; these casualties had no other injuries.

    h. The use of temporary tourniquets to stop the bleeding is essential in these types of casualties. If the casualty needs to be moved, as is usually the case, a tourniquet is the most reasonable initial choice to stop major bleeding. Ischemic damage to the limb is rare if the tourniquet is left in place for less than one hour (tourniquets are often left in place for several hours during surgical procedures). In addition, the use of a temporary tourniquet may allow the injured soldier to continue to fight. Both the casualty and the soldier medic are in grave danger while applying the tourniquet and non-life-threatening bleeding should be ignored until the tactical field care phase.

i.   The need for immediate access to a tourniquet in such situations makes it clear that all soldiers on combat missions have a suitable tourniquet, such as the Combat Application Tourniquet (CAT) shown in figure 1-2, readily available at a standard location on their battle gear and that soldiers be trained in its use.

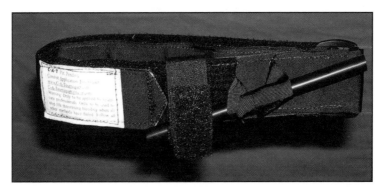

Figure 1-2. The Combat Application Tourniquet (CAT).

j.   Penetrating neck injuries do not require cervical spine (C-spine) immobilization. Other neck injuries, such as falls over 15 feet, fast roping injuries, or motor vehicle collisions (MVC), may require C-spine immobilization unless the danger of hostile fire constitutes a greater threat in the judgment of the soldier medic. Studies have shown that, with penetrating neck injuries being only 1.4 percent of the injured, few would have benefited from C-spine immobilization. Adjustable rigid cervical colors (C-collars) should be carried in the soldier medic's medical aid bag. If rigid C-collars are not available, a SAM splint from the aid bag can be used as a field expedient C-collar.

k.   Litters may not be available for movement of casualties.

(1)   Consider alternate methods to move casualties, such as ponchos, pole-less litters, SKEDCO or Talon II litters, discarded doors, dragging, or manual carries).

(2)   Smoke, CS (2-chlorobenzalmalononitrile, a type of riot control gas), and vehicles may act as screens to assist in casualty movement.

l.   Do not attempt to salvage a casualty's rucksack unless it contains items critical to the mission. Take the casualty's weapon and ammunition, if possible, to prevent the enemy from using them against you.

m. Key points.

    (1)   Return fire as directed or required.

    (2)   The casualty should also return fire if able.

    (3)   Direct the casualty to cover and apply self-aid, if able.

    (4)   Try to keep the casualty from sustaining any additional wounds.

    (5)   Airway management is generally best deferred until the tactical field care phase.

    (6)   Stop any life-threatening hemorrhage with a tourniquet or a HemCon™ Bandage, if applicable.

1-4. TACTICAL FIELD CARE

The "tactical field care" phase is distinguished from the "care under fire" phase by having more time available to provide care and a reduced level of hazard from hostile fire.

a. The time available to render care may be quite variable. In some cases, tactical field care may consist of rapid treatment of wounds with the expectation of a re-engagement of hostile fire at any moment. In some circumstances, there may be ample time to render whatever care is available in the field. The time to evacuation may be quite variable from minutes to several hours.

b. If a victim of a blast or penetrating injury is found without a pulse, respirations, or other signs of life, do not attempt cardiopulmonary resuscitation (CPR). Attempts to resuscitate trauma casualties in arrest have found to be futile even in the urban setting where the victim is in close proximity to a trauma center. On the battlefield, the cost of attempting CPR on casualties with what are inevitably fatal injuries will be measured in additional lives lost as care is withheld from casualties with less severe injuries and as soldier medics are exposed to additional hazard from hostile fire because of their attempts. Only in the case of non-traumatic disorders, such as hypothermia, near drowning, or electrocution, should CPR be considered. Casualties with an altered level of consciousness should be disarmed immediately. Remove both weapons and grenades. This provides a safety measure for the care providers. When the casualty becomes more awake and alert he could mistake the good guys for the enemy he was recently engaging.

c. Initial assessment consists of airway, breathing, and circulation.

d. Oxygen is usually not available in this phase. Cylinders of compressed gas and the associated equipment for supplying the oxygen are too heavy to make their use in the field feasible.

e. Breathing.

(1) Traumatic chest wall defects should be closed with an occlusive dressing without regard to venting one side of the dressing, as this is difficult to do in a combat setting. You may use an Asherman chest seal (lesson 3) if one is available.

(2) If you are taping a field dressing envelope or other airtight material over an open chest wound, tape all four sides of the material to the chest as long as the care provider has the ability to needle decompress a possible tension pneumothorax. If the ability to needle decompress the chest is not available, the occlusive dressing should only be taped on three sides to allow a flutter valve effect in the dressing.

NOTE: Tension pneumothorax is the second leading cause of preventable battlefield death.

f. Bleeding.

(1) The soldier medic should now address any significant bleeding sites not previously controlled. He should only remove the absolute minimum of clothing required to expose and treat injuries, both because of time constraints and the need to protect the patient from environmental extremes.

(2) Significant bleeding should be stopped as quickly as possible using a tourniquet as described previously. Once the tactical situation permits, consideration should be given to loosening the tourniquet and using direct pressure, a pressure dressing, a chitosan hemostatic dressing, or a hemostatic powder (QuikClot) to control any additional hemorrhage. Do not completely remove the tourniquet, just loosen it and leave in place. If hemorrhage continues, the tourniquet should be retightened and left alone.

g. Intravenous access.

NOTE: Intravenous infusion procedures are discussed in MD0553, Intravenous Infusions and Related Tasks.

(1) Intravenous access should be gained next. Although advanced trauma life support (ATLS) recommends starting two large-bore (14- or 16- gauge) intravenous infusions (IVs), the use of a single 18-gauge catheter is preferred in the field setting because of the ease of starting the infusions and because it also serves to ration supplies.

(2)   Heparin or saline lock-type access tubing should be used unless the patient needs immediate fluid resuscitation. Flushing the saline lock every two hours will usually suffice to keep it open without the need to use a heparin solution.

(3)   Soldier medics should ensure the IV is not started distal to a significant wound.

(4)   If you are unable to initiate a peripheral IV, consideration should be given to starting a sternal intraosseous (IO) line to provide fluids. When unable to gain vascular access through a peripheral vein, an IO device can be used to gain access through the sternum. The First Access for Shock and Trauma (F.A.S.T.1) device is available and allows the puncture of the manubrium of the sternum and administration of fluids at rates similar to IVs. See figure 1-3.

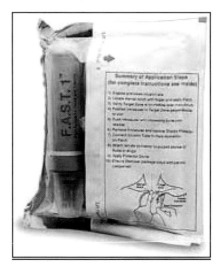

Figure 1-3. The F.A.S.T.1.

h. Intravenous fluids.

(1)   One thousand milliliters (ml) of Ringer's lactate (2.4 pounds) will expand the intravascular volume 250 ml within one hour.

(2)   Five hundred ml of 6 percent hetastarch (trade name Hextend®) weighs 1.3 pounds and will expand the intravascular volume by 800 ml within one hour. One 500 ml bag of Hextend® solution is functionally equivalent to three 1,000 ml bags of lactated Ringer's. There is more than a 5 1/2 pound advantage in the overall weight-to-benefit ratio (1.3 lbs to 7.2 lbs, respectively). The expansion using Hextend® is sustained for at least eight hours. For these reasons, Hextend® is the fluid of choice. See figure 1-4 for an illustration of an IV bag of Hextend®.

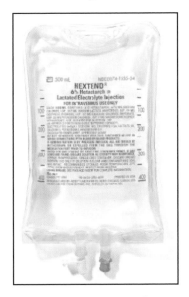

Figure 1-4. Hextend®.

(3)   The first consideration in selecting a resuscitation fluid is whether to use a crystalloid or colloid solution. Crystalloids are fluids such as Ringer's lactate or normal saline where sodium is the primary osmotically-active solute. Since sodium eventually distributes throughout the entire extracellular space, most of the fluids in crystalloid solutions remain in the intravascular space for only a limited time. Colloids such as Hextend® are solutions where the primary osmotically active molecules are of greater molecular weight and do not readily pass through the capillary walls into the interstitial space. These solutions are retained in the intravascular space for a much longer period than crystalloids. In addition, the oncotic pressure of colloid solutions may result in an expansion of the blood volume that is greater than the amount infused.

i. Any significant extremity or truncal wound (neck, chest, abdomen, and pelvis), with or without obvious blood loss or hypotension, may require intravenous infusion.

(1) If the casualty is coherent and has a palpable radial pulse, blood loss has likely stopped. Initiate a saline lock, hold fluids, and re-evaluate as frequently as the situation allows.

(2) If there is significant blood loss from any wound and the casualty has no radial pulse or is not coherent, <u>STOP THE BLEEDING</u> by whatever means available (tourniquet, direct pressure, hemostatic dressing [HemCon™], or hemostatic powder [QuikClot]). However, greater than 90 percent of hypotensive casualties suffer from truncal injuries that are not corrected by these resuscitative measures. These casualties will have lost a minimum of 1,500 ml of blood (30 percent of their circulating volume). After hemorrhage is controlled to the extent possible, start 500 ml of Hextend®. If mental status improves and the radial pulse returns, maintain the saline lock and hold fluids.

(3) If no response is seen, within 30 minutes, give an additional 500 ml. of Hextend® and monitor vital signs. If no response is seen after 1,000 ml of Hextend®, consider triaging supplies and giving attention to more salvageable casualties. Remember, this amount is equivalent to more than 6 liters of Ringer's lactate.

(4) Because of the need to conserve existing supplies, no casualty should receive more than 1,000 ml of Hextend®.

(5) Uncontrolled thoracic or intra-abdominal hemorrhage needs rapid evacuation and surgical intervention. If this is not possible, determine the number of casualties verses the amount of available fluids. If supplies are limited or casualties are numerous, determine if fluid resuscitation is recommended.

NOTE: A number of studies involving uncontrolled hemorrhage models have clearly established that aggressive fluid resuscitation in the setting of unrepaired vascular injury is either of no benefit or results in an increase in blood loss and/or mortality when compared to no fluid resuscitation or hypotensive resuscitation. Several studies noted that only after uncontrolled hemorrhage was stopped did fluid resuscitation prove to be of benefit.

j. Dress wounds to prevent further contamination and help hemostasis. Emergency trauma dressings (Israeli bandages) are ideal for this. Check for additional wounds (exit wounds) since the high velocity projectiles from modern assault rifles may tumble and take erratic courses when traveling through tissues, often leading to exit sites that are remote from the entry wound.

k. Only remove enough clothing to expose and treat wounds. Care must be taken to protect the casualty from hypothermia. Casualties who are hypovolemic become hypothermic quite rapidly if traveling in a CASEVAC or MEDEVAC asset and are not protected from the wind, regardless of the ambient temperature. Protect the casualty by wrapping them in a protective wrap (Blizzard Rescue Wrap®)

l. Pain control.

(1) If the casualty is able to fight, administer meloxicam (Mobic™) 15 milligrams (mg) taken orally (PO) initially with two 650 mg of acetominophen (bi-layered Tylenol® caplets) every eight hours. Along with an antibiotic, this makes up the "combat pill pack" depicted figure 1-5.

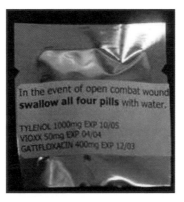

Figure 1-5. Combat pill pack.

(2) If the casualty is unable to fight, 5 mg IV morphine may be given every 10 minutes until adequate pain control is achieved. If a saline lock is used, it should be flushed with 5 ml of saline after the morphine administration. Ensure there is some visible indication of time and amount of morphine given. Document the morphine administration on the casualty's field medical card (FMC).

m. Fractures should be splinted as circumstances allow. Perform pulse, motor, and sensory (PMS) checks before and after splinting.

n. Antibiotics should be considered in all battlefield wounds since these type wounds are prone to infection. Infection is a late cause of morbidity and mortality in wounds sustained on the battlefield.

o. Combat is a frightening experience, especially if wounded. Reassure the casualty. This can be simply telling him that you are there and are going to take care of him. It can be as effective as morphing in relieving anxiety. Explain the care that is being given.

p. Document clinical assessments, treatment rendered, and changes in the casualty's status. Forward the documentation with the casualty to next level of care.

1-5. CASUALTY EVACUATION CARE

a. At some point in the operation, the casualty will be scheduled for evacuation. However, evacuation time may be quite variable, from minutes to hours to days. There are a multitude of factors that will affect the ability to evacuate a casualty. Availability of aircraft or vehicles, weather, tactical situation, and mission may all reflect the ability or inability to evacuate casualties.

b. There are only minor differences in the care provided in the CASEVAC phase verses the tactical field care phase.

(1) Additional medical personnel may accompany the evacuation asset and assist the soldier medic on the ground. This may be important for the following reasons:

(a) The soldier medic may be among the casualties.

(b) The soldier medic may be dehydrated, hypothermic or otherwise debilitated.

(c) The evacuation asset's medical equipment may need to be prepared prior to evacuation.

(d) There may be multiple casualties that exceed the capability of the soldier medic to care for simultaneously.

(2) Additional medical equipment can be brought with the evacuation asset to augment the equipment the soldier medic currently has. This equipment may include:

(a) Electronic monitoring equipment capable of measuring a casualty's blood pressure, pulse, and pulse oximetry (oxygen saturation of the arterial blood).

(b) Oxygen should be available during this phase.

(c) Ringer's lactate at a rate of 250 ml per hour for casualties that are not in shock should help to reverse dehydration, and in some special circumstances blood products may be available during this phase.

(d) Thermal Angel fluid warmers may be needed to warm IV fluids.

(e) A pneumatic anti-shock garment (PASG), if available, may be beneficial in pelvic fractures and helping to control pelvic and abdominal bleeding. The PASG is contraindicated in thoracic and traumatic brain injuries).

Continue with Exercises

EXERCISES, LESSON 1

INSTRUCTIONS: Answer the following exercises by marking the lettered response that best answers the question or best completes the sentence or by writing the answer in the space provided.

After you have answered all of the exercises, turn to "Solutions to Exercises" at the end of the lesson and check your answers. For each exercise answered incorrectly, reread the lesson material referenced with the solution.

1. List the three phase in tactical combat casualty care.

    _____

    _____

    _____

2. What is the primary source of hemorrhage control during the care under fire phase?

    a. Direct pressure.

    b. Elevation.

    c. Pressure points.

    d. Tourniquet.

3. You have moved your casualty to a collection point where the casualty has been loaded into a ground ambulance. What stage of TC3 are you in?

    a. Care under fire.

    b. Tactical field care.

    c. CASEVAC care.

4. What is your first concern during care under fire?

   a. Providing care for a wounded soldier.

   b. Continue the mission.

   c. Recovering non-essential equipment.

   d. Gaining fire superiority.

5. You have multiple casualties. Casualty A has minor wounds; Casualty B has major injuries; and Casualty C is in cardiopulmonary arrest due to massive blood loss. You are the only medic available. What is your best course of action?

   a. Begin CPR on casualty C.

   b. Triage your supplies and casualties; treat casualty B.

   c. Wait until more help arrives.

6. Intravenous access should be gained during which phase of TC3?

   a. Care under fire.

   b. Tactical field care.

   c. CASEVAC care.

7. Two large bore IVs wide open should be started for all casualties.

   a. True.

   b. False.

8. The fluid of choice for hypovolemic fluid resuscitation is:

   a. Normal saline.

   b. Five percent dextrose in water.

   c. Ringer's lactate.

   d. Hextend®.

9. If unable to obtain a patent peripheral IV what is the next option?

   a. Package the patient for transport.

   b. F.A.S.T.1 intra-osseous

   c. Intravenous cut down

10. Which of the following is NOT additional medical equipment that can be brought in during the CASEVAC phase of care?

   a. Electronic monitoring equipment capable of measuring a casualty's blood pressure, pulse and pulse oximetry.

   b. Oxygen

   c. Field surgical table to perform needed surgeries at the point of injury.

   d. Thermal Angel fluid warmers to warm IV fluids.

Check Your Answers on Next Page

SOLUTIONS TO EXERCISES, LESSON 1

1. Care under fire
    Tactical field care
    CASEVAC care   (paras 1-1; 1-2a, b, c)

2. d   (para 1-3h)

3. c   (para1-2c)

4. d   (para 1-3a)

5. b   (para 1-4b)

6. c   (para 1-4g)

7. b   (para 1-4g(1))

8. d   (para 1-4h(2))

9. b   (para 1-4g(4))

10. c   (para 1-5b(2))

End of Lesson 1

LESSON ASSIGNMENT

LESSON 2   Controlling Bleeding From an Extremity.

TEXT ASSIGNMENT   Paragraphs 2-1 through 2-35.

LESSON OBJECTIVES   When you have completed this lesson, you should be able to:

2-1.   Identify the procedures for applying a field dressing to a wound.

2-2.   Identify the procedures for applying manual pressure and elevation to a wound.

2-3.   Identify the procedures for applying a pressure dressing to a wound.

2-4.   Identify pressure points used to control bleeding.

2-5.   Identify the procedures for applying a tourniquet.

2-6.   Identify the procedures for treating an amputation.

2-7.   Identify the procedures for treating a limb with internal bleeding.

SUGGESTION   Work the lesson exercises at the end of this lesson before beginning the next lesson. These exercises will help you accomplish the lesson objectives.

LESSON 2

CONTROLLING BLEEDING FROM AN EXTREMITY

Section I. GENERAL

2-1. HYPOVOLEMIC SHOCK

Blood supplies the brain and other body parts with the oxygen and nutrients they need to live and function. A sudden decrease in the amount of blood in the circulatory system, such as that caused by severe bleeding, endangers these tissues. A sudden decrease in blood volume can also produce hypovolemic (low volume) shock. An average adult has about six quarts (around 5000 to 6000 milliliters) of blood in his body.

a. Blood products can not be replaced on the front line of the battlefield, so it must be stopped at all costs. The old school of thought of treating with direct pressure and then elevation and working your way to a tourniquet as a last resort is antiquated. Modern medical research has proven that on the battlefield lives will be saved with the aggressive use of tourniquets and then attempting to reduce these to pressure dressings as the situation permits.

b. Figure 2-1 shows the effects of blood loss on the body. This guide can help you determine the amount of loss the patient has already suffered. Once the patient has reached stages III and IV, it is often too late. This helps to demonstrate the importance of early and aggressive control of hemorrhage on the battlefield.

Class	Blood Loss	Clinical Signs
I	Up to 750 ml (15 percent)	Slight increase in heart rate; no change in blood pressure or respirations
II	750 to 1500 ml (15 to 30 percent)	Increased heart rate and respirations; increased diastolic blood pressure; anxiety, fright or hostility
III	1500 to 2000 ml (30 to 40 percent)	Increased heart rate and respirations; fall in systolic blood pressure; significant AMS
IV	Over 2000 ml (over 40 percent)	Severe tachycardia; severe lowering of blood pressure; cold, pale skin; severe AMS

NOTE: Altered mental status (AMS).

Figure 2-1. Effects of blood loss.

2-2. EXTERNAL AND INTERNAL BLEEDING

Serious bleeding (hemorrhage) usually results when an artery or vein is cut or torn (such as being punctured by shrapnel or the sharp end of a fractured bone) or when the blood vessel is ruptured due to disease or a blow with a blunt instrument. Bleeding may be either external or internal.

a. **External Bleeding.** When the bleeding is external, blood can be seen coming from an open (skin is broken) wound. External bleeding can be from an artery (a blood vessel which carries blood away from the heart), from a vein (a blood vessel which carries blood back to the heart), or from capillaries (tiny blood vessels connecting an artery and a vein).

(1) Arterial blood is bright red (rich in oxygen) and is usually expelled from the wound in spurts. The spurts are caused by the pulse waves resulting from the heart's pumping actions (contractions).

(2) Venous blood is a dark bluish-red (low in oxygen content) and flows at a slower, steady rate. Venous blood does not escape in spurts because the pulse is not present in the veins.

(3) Capillary blood resembles venous blood in color. The very small size of capillaries causes the escaping blood to ooze from a wound rather than flow at a more rapid rate.

b. **Internal Bleeding.** Internal bleeding occurs when the blood from a damaged blood vessel or organ (such as a laceration of the liver) flows into a body cavity or is trapped in the surrounding tissue rather than escaping the body through an open wound. Internal bleeding can be identified by discolored tissue (bruises), swelling (from blood escaping into surrounding tissue), rigid body cavity (cavity filled with blood), and/or blood escaping through a body orifice such as the mouth, rectum, or vagina. The casualty may cough up blood (hemoptysis), vomit blood (hematemesis), or pass bloody stools (hematochezia). Vomited blood may be bright red or it may be dark and resemble coffee grounds. The stools may be bright red or dark (melena). Blood loss from internal bleeding is just as serious as visible blood loss from external bleeding.

2-3. NATURAL BODY REACTIONS TO BLEEDING

The body has natural mechanisms that act to control bleeding.

a. **Contraction.** If a blood vessel is severed, the end of the vessel may contract and decrease the size of the opening through which blood can escape the vessel. This contraction is temporary and full bleeding will occur when the vessel relaxes. Contraction can often lead to a false impression of the severity of the wound. During care under fire, aggressive use of tourniquets is needed to ensure that, as the body starts to relax, the patient does not bleed out.

b. **Clotting.** The body's primary defense against blood loss is clotting. When a blood vessel is damaged or cut, platelets (thrombocytes) in the blood attach themselves to the damaged part of the blood vessel and begin plugging the opening. Fibrinogen in the blood changes to fibrin and reinforces the platelets. An insoluble clot forms that plugs the torn or cut blood vessel until the vessel is repaired. If the blood vessel is large and the damage is severe, a clot may not form in time to stop the bleeding.

c. **Immobilization.** The body may also react to damage by immobilizing the injured part. The casualty with an injured leg may fall or lie down and remain still. The muscles become more rigid to decrease pain and the casualty will tend to avoid moving the injured body part. This natural splinting reaction helps to reduce blood loss by restricting activity of the body part. The more active the body part, the greater the blood flow in the injured part.

2-4. COMMONLY USED TERMS

a. **Signs and Symptoms.** A sign is something the medic can detect, such as seeing a bruise, hearing noises during breathing, or measuring vital signs. A symptom is a complaint voiced by the casualty that the medic cannot directly observe, such as pain in the casualty's back or a headache.

b. **Dressing.** The term dressing refers to the material that is placed directly on top of the open wound. The dressing absorbs some of the blood and helps a clot to form. The clot, if successful, plugs the opening in the blood vessel and stops the bleeding. The dressing also protects the wound from additional contamination and injury. A dressing can be applied to any open wound.

c. **Bandage.** A bandage is the material used to hold (secure) the dressing in place so the dressing will not slip and destroy the clot that is forming. In addition to keeping the dressing in place, the pressure applied by the bandage also helps to compress the injured blood vessel and, thereby, reduce bleeding. The ends of the bandage are called the tails.

d. **Field Dressing.** The field dressing (also called the field first aid dressing or bandage or the combat dressing) consists of a pad of sterile (germ-free) white dressing with a bandage (usually olive-drab) already attached to the dressing pad (figure 2-2). The field dressing is wrapped in paper which is then sealed in a plastic envelope. The field dressing is starting to be replaced by the emergency trauma dressing discussed below.

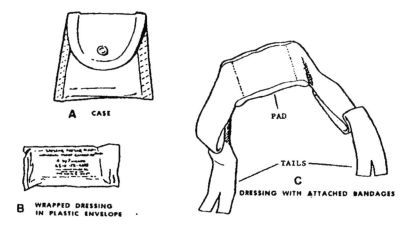

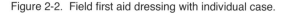

Figure 2-2. Field first aid dressing with individual case.

e. **Emergency Trauma Dressing**. The emergency trauma dressing, sometimes called the "Israeli dressing," is a combination dressing and compression bandage that incorporates a pressure applying locking bar and elastic bandage (figure 2-3). This allows a great deal of pressure to be applied directly to the wound. The emergency trauma dressing has a thin, sterile non-adherent pad with a tan elastic bandage attached to the dressing. The emergency trauma dressing is part of the improved first aid kit (figure 2-4) that is replacing the first aid kit shown in figure 2-2.

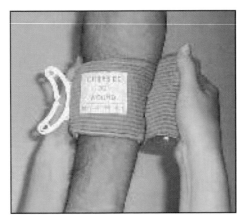

Figure 2-3 Emergency trauma dressing.

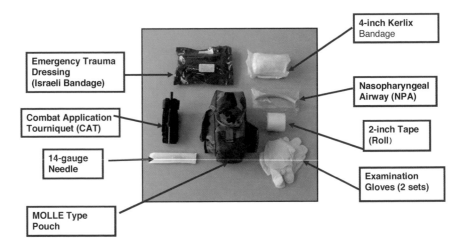

NOTE: The 14-gauge needle will only be carried by qualified personnel.

Figure 2-4. Improved first aid kit (weight 1.08 pounds; cube 128 cubic inches).

f. **Pressure Dressing.** A pressure dressing consists of a wad of material placed over a regular dressing and secured with a tight bandage. The pressure dressing is used to apply continuous pressure on the wound in an effort to compress blood vessels and help control bleeding. The pressure dressing does not stop the flow of blood through arteries and veins. A pressure dressing is only applied to a wound on a limb (arm or leg).

f. **Pressure Point.** A pressure point is a place on the body where an artery lies near the skin surface and passes over a bony area. Blood flow through the artery can be stopped by pressing on the artery at such a point. The artery, trapped between the bone and the pressure, collapses and blood cannot get through. Pressure points are not recommended on the battlefield when a tourniquet would be more appropriate since the tourniquet does not require the medic to dedicate his attention to applying pressure.

g. **Tourniquet.** A tourniquet is a band placed around the upper arm, forearm, thigh, or lower leg that stops the flow of the blood below (distal to) the band. A tourniquet is the treatment of choice during the care under fire phase of battle. During subsequent phases of care, the tourniquet will be assessed for removal (it may be kept in place if required).

(1) The limb below the level of the tourniquet may have to be amputated. However, tourniquets used in surgery to stop the blood flow to a limb are left in place for up to two hours without complications. If the casualty is allowed to continue bleeding, he will die. Therefore, the benefit of the tourniquet outweighs the potential risk to the casualty.

(2) Current research has proven that aggressive early use of tourniquets saves lives.

(3) It is the goal that every soldier has a tourniquet available and knows how to use it. Manufactured tourniquets such as the Combat Application Tourniquet (CAT) are great for meeting this goal. (See figure 2-5.) The combat medic should never forget that improvised tourniquets are still sound medical equipment and should be available to supplement manufactured tourniquets. (See figure 2-6.)

NOTE: Keep in mind the number of tourniquets that may be required at a moment's notice. A HMMWV (high mobility multi-purpose wheeled vehicle) with a gunner can carry five personnel. That means that 20 tourniquets could be needed. Even with every soldier carrying a tourniquet, they may not be readily available to the combat medic under fire.

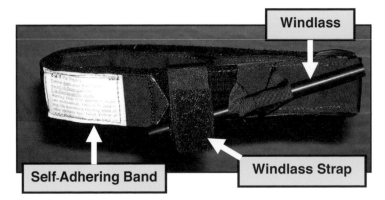

Figure 2-5. The Combat Application Tourniquet (CAT).

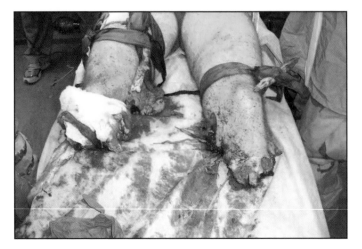

Figure 2-6. Properly used Improvised tourniquets.

2-5. METHODS OF CONTROLLING BLEEDING

During the care under fire phase, the first thing you should look for is significant bleeding. If you are in doubt of the significance of the bleed, apply a tourniquet immediately and assess it later when you have more time. The body's natural mechanisms may not be able to control the bleeding. A casualty who is losing blood rapidly may die unless the bleeding is stopped. When severe bleeding is discovered, stop your survey and take measures to control bleeding.

NOTE: This lesson is concerned with controlling bleeding from an extremity.
Bleeding from the trunk and from the head is covered in other lessons.

a. External bleeding will be controlled initially with a tourniquet during care
under fire. Once the medic has transitioned to the tactical field care phase, the
tourniquet will be evaluated for need in the following manner.

(1)   If the bleeding seems significant (venous or arterial), then a tourniquet
should be applied during the care under fire phase.

(2)   The tourniquet can be loosened during the care under fire phase under
the following conditions.

(a)   Based on the tactical situation. When there is a lull in the battle or
the battle has moved away from the casualty collection point.

(b)   More time in a safer setting. You have enough time and
protection to assess the need for a tourniquet and reapply it if you determine that it is
still needed.

(c)   More help is available. Additional hands may be needed to
assess and reapply the tourniquet.

(3)   If you are unable to control bleeding with other methods, retighten the
tourniquet. The need to prevent further blood loss is greater than the potential risks
associated with tourniquet application.

(4)   Some other considerations involving tourniquets are given below.

(a)   Can you see what you are doing? Enough light is essential to
adequately assess the bleeding.

(b)   Does the casualty need fluid resuscitation? If so, do it before the
tourniquet is removed. Ensure a positive response is obtained; that is, the casualty
has good peripheral pulse and good mentation (mental ability).

(c)   DO NOT periodically loosen the tourniquet to get blood to the
limb. This is an antiquated technique that will only cause the casualty to lose more
blood that can not be replaced on the front lines.

(d)   Tourniquets are very painful. It has been documented that
patients have tried to remove tourniquets due to the pain they cause. Be prepared to
administer narcotic analgesic pain control to casualties to protect them and to provide
for their comfort.

(e)   If the tourniquet has been on for more than six hours, leave it on. At this point, do not attempt to remove the tourniquet.

b. Once in the tactical field care phase, any bleeding not previously treated should be assessed and treated.

(1)   Application of emergency trauma dressings, hemostatic agents, or other means to control simple bleeding may be used at this time.

(2)   Hemostatic dressings contain an agent to aid in the clotting process. Currently the Army has approved the HemCon™ Bandage (figure 2-7) for use on the battlefield. Other agents are in existence, but are not currently approved by the Army. The HemCon dressing contains an agent that is non-allergenic and is readily absorbed by the body during the healing process. This agent speeds the clotting process when it is applied directly to the wound. This dressing is advised for bleeding that can not be controlled by tourniquets or other direct pressure, such as high femoral bleeding or truncal bleeding.

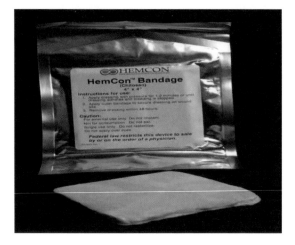

Figure 2-7. Hem-Con™ hemostatic dressing.

Section II. CONTROLLING EXTERNAL BLEEDING FROM A WOUND ON AN EXTREMITY

2-6. LOCATE THE WOUND

Look and feel for amputations, bloody clothing, wounds, and pools of blood. If the bleeding is severe enough to threaten the casualty's life (heavy bleeding from an artery or a large vein or bleeding from a major amputation), treat it as soon as it is discovered. Less serious bleeding can be controlled during the tactical field care phase.

2-7. EXPOSE THE WOUND

After locating the wound area, fully expose the wound so you can see the full extent of the injury. Tear, cut, push, or lift the casualty's clothing from the area. Some special considerations are given in the following paragraphs.

a. **Care Under Fire.** Expose only the area necessary to apply a tourniquet during this phase.

b. **Tactical Field Care.** Expose the area to fully evaluate the wound and assess further for entry and exit wounds. Be aware that you and the casualty may still be at risk of re-engagement by the enemy and the casualty may need his body armor. Hypothermia is also a major consideration even in extreme heat. With loss of blood, the casualty's body may not be able to compensate. Appropriate steps should be taken to prevent hypothermia since hypothermia also inhibits the clotting process.

c. **Chemical Environment.** If you are in a chemical environment (chemical agents present), do not expose the wound since this would increase the casualty's exposure to the chemical agents. Apply a tourniquet or place a field dressing over the wound and clothing and secure with the attached bandages, as appropriate. Evacuate the casualty as soon as possible.

e. **Spinal Injury.** If you suspect the casualty has a spinal injury, use scissors from your aid bag to cut the clothing rather than tearing it. Cutting the clothing keeps movement of the casualty to a minimum.

f. **Fractured Limb.** If the bleeding is from a limb and you suspect the limb is fractured (limb in an abnormal position), use scissors to cut the clothing to keep movement of the limb to a minimum.

g. **Entry and Exit Wounds.** Look for both an entry wound and an exit wound. If more than one wound is found, treat the more serious wound (the wound that is bleeding the most or the larger wound) first.

h. **Stuck Material.** If clothing or other material is stuck to the wound area, cut or tear around the stuck material. This frees the other material while leaving the material stuck to the wound. Do not pull the stuck material from the wound since removing the material might cause additional damage to the wound. Apply the dressing over the stuck material.

i. **Debris in Wound.** Do not remove objects from the wound. Do not probe the wound in an attempt to locate a missile (such as a bullet or piece of shrapnel) that may be lodged in the wound. Objects that protrude from the wound should be stabilized with bulky dressings.

2-8. CHECK THE CIRCULATION BELOW THE WOUND

Check the casualty's blood circulation and nerve function distal to (below) the wound during the tactical field care phase. If possible, compare the area below the wound to the same area on the uninjured limb. If a pulse cannot be felt below the wound or other indications of impairment are present, evacuate the casualty as soon as possible after life-saving procedures have been completed in order to save the limb. Assume that blood circulation and/or nerve function below the wound is impaired if:

a. There is no pulse below the wound or the pulse is weaker than the pulse in the uninjured limb.

b. The skin and/or nail beds below the wound are bluish (cyanosis).

c. The skin below the wound is cooler to the touch than the same area on the uninjured limb.

d. The portion of the limb below the wound is numb or has decreased sensation when compared to the same area on the uninjured limb. (The casualty must be conscious and able to think clearly in order to make this test.)

e. Motor function of the limb below the wound is lost. (The casualty must be conscious and able to think clearly in order to verify that he cannot move his hand and fingers or cannot move his feet and toes.)

2-9. APPLY AND SECURE THE FIELD DRESSING

NOTE: This paragraph assumes that you have a field first-aid dressing and will apply it to an open wound.

After you have exposed the wound and checked the circulation, apply the field dressing to the wound and secure the dressing using the following procedures.

a. **Obtain a Field Dressing.**

(1)   If the soldier has a field dressing in his plastic individual first aid case, use his field dressing in order to conserve your supplies. If he does not have a field dressing available, use a field dressing from your aid bag.

(2)   If the wound is large, you may need to improvise a dressing and bandage from the cleanest materials available.

b. **Remove the Field Dressing From the Wrappers.**

(1)   Locate the notch (slit) in one end of the plastic envelope containing the field dressing.

(2)   Beginning at the notch, tear the plastic envelope open and remove the inner packet. The packet is the field dressing in a paper wrapper. Discard the plastic envelope (unless you need it to seal an open chest wound as described in Lesson 3).

(3)   Grasp the packet with both hands and twist until the paper wrapper breaks.

(4)   Remove the field dressing from the paper wrapper and discard the paper wrapper. Avoid touching the white dressing pad of the field dressing. The pad is sterile and should be kept as free from contamination as possible. Hold on to the tails only.

c. **Apply the Dressing to the Wound.**

(1)   Grasp the folded tails of the field dressing with both hands (figure 2-8 A.)

(2)   Hold the field dressing above the exposed wound with the sterile pad of dressing material toward the wound.

(3)   Pull on the tails so the dressing opens and flattens (figure 2-8 B).

(4)   Place the white dressing pad directly on the wound (figures 2-8 C and D).

A

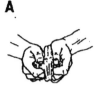

PREPARE TO OPEN DRESSING.

B

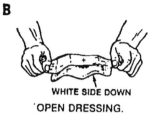

WHITE SIDE DOWN

OPEN DRESSING.

C   **D**

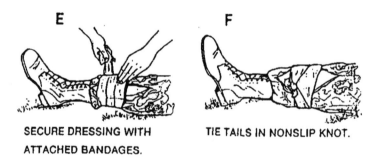

APPLY DRESSING TO WOUND.

E   **F**

SECURE DRESSING WITH   TIE TAILS IN NONSLIP KNOT.
ATTACHED BANDAGES.

Figure 2-8. Applying and securing a field dressing to a wound on a leg.

(a)   If an object (piece of shrapnel, twig from a tree or bush, or such) is protruding from the wound, apply dressings to the wound without covering the protruding object. Procedures for dressing a wound with a protruding object are given in Lesson 8 of this subcourse.

(b)   If the fractured end of a bone can be seen, cover the bone with the dressing. Do not attempt to force the bone beneath the skin. Do not attempt to realign the fractured limb.

d. **Secure the Dressing.**

(1)   Place one hand on top of the dressing to hold the dressing in place and to apply pressure to the bleeding blood vessels. If the casualty is conscious, you can have him apply pressure to the dressing while you secure it.

(2)   Wrap one of the bandages around the injured limb with your free hand. As you wrap, cover one of the exposed sides of the dressing with the bandage. (The bandage can usually be wrapped around a limb more than once.) Bring the tail back over the dressing.

(3)   Wrap the other bandage around the injured body part in the opposite direction (figure 2-8 E). As you wrap, cover the remaining exposed side of the dressing with the bandage. Bring the tail back to the dressing.

(4)   Tie the tails in a non-slip knot at the edge of the dressing (figure 2-8 F).

2-10. CHECK THE CIRCULATION BELOW THE FIELD DRESSING

Recheck the casualty's blood circulation and nerve function below the wound. The blood circulation and/or nerve function is impaired if the pulse below the limb is absent or impaired, if the skin or nail beds below the wound are bluish, if the limb below the wound is numb or cool to the touch, or if motor function below the wound is lost. If possible, compare the area below the wound of the injured limb to the same area on the uninjured limb. If the circulation or nerve function is impaired, loosen the tails with disturbing the dressing and retie the tails. If circulation and nerve function are not restored, evacuate the casualty as soon as possible.

2-11. ELEVATE THE INJURED LIMB, IF APPROPRIATE

a. **Check for a Fracture.** Examine the injured limb for fractures (visible broken bone, deformity of the limb, and such). If a fracture is suspected, do not elevate the wound at this time. If a fractured limb is moved before a splint is applied, the sharp edges of the fractured bone may damage nearby nerves and blood vessels. A fractured limb can be elevated after a splint has been applied to the fractured limb.

b. **Elevate the Limb.** If the injured limb is not fractured (or if a splint has already been applied) and the limb does not have an impaled (protruding) object, raise the limb above the level of the casualty's heart. Elevating the limb will help to decrease blood flow to the injured area and, thereby, reduce bleeding and swelling. Make sure the limb is supported and the limb will not slip off the support. Elevating the injured limb and applying manual pressure should be done at the same time when no fracture is involved.

(1)   If the wound is on a leg, place a pack, log, rock, or other object under the foot and ankle of the injured leg (figure 2-9).

(2)   If the wound is on an arm and the casualty is lying on his back, place the casualty's forearm on his chest.

(3)   If wound is on an arm and the casualty is sitting up, have the casualty place his forearm on top of his head.

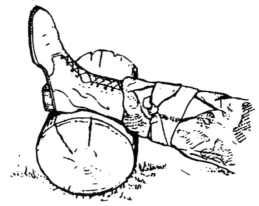

Figure 2-9. Elevating a wound on a leg.

2-12. RE-EVALUATE THE BLEEDING

After the field dressing, manual pressure, and elevation (if appropriate) have been applied, check the dressing to see if the bleeding has been controlled.

a. If the dressing is saturated with blood and fresh (red) blood is seeping out of the dressing, the bleeding has not been adequately controlled. If the bleeding is not controlled by this point consideration of a tourniquet or hemostatic dressing is necessary to prevent further bleeding.

b. If the bleeding has been controlled, continue your evaluation.

(1) If the dressing is saturated with blood, additional dressing material may be applied on top of the field dressing and secured with bandages (muslin bandage, roller bandage, or torn strips of material). Do not remove the field dressing or disturb any clots that have formed.

(2) Monitor the casualty. If bleeding begins again, evaluate the bleeding and apply a pressure dressing if needed.

2-13. APPLY DIGITAL PRESSURE, IF NEEDED

If an artery is damaged, you can use your finger, thumb, hand, or knee to apply pressure to the artery at a pressure point above the wound. The pressure compresses the artery against the bone, thus reducing blood flow or stopping the blood flow entirely. Since it is difficult to maintain sufficient pressure on the artery and more than one blood vessel is usually involved in the injury, the pressure point method is used only until a pressure dressing can be applied. Figure 2-10 shows the location of common pressure points. A pulse can always be felt at a pressure point.

a. To control arterial bleeding of the upper part of the upper arm, apply pressure to the subclavian artery (figure 2-10 D).

b. To control arterial bleeding of the lower part of the upper arm or at the elbow, apply pressure to the brachial artery (figure 2-10 E).

c. To control arterial bleeding of the forearm, apply pressure to the lower part of the brachial artery (figure 2-10 F) or to the ulnar or radial artery.

d. To control arterial bleeding of the wrist or hand, apply pressure to the ulnar or radial artery (figure 2-10 G).

e. To control arterial bleeding of the thigh, apply pressure to the femoral artery (figures 2-10 H and I).

f. To control arterial bleeding of the lower leg, apply pressure to the popliteal artery (figure 2-10 J).

g. To control arterial bleeding of the foot, apply pressure to the anterior or posterior tibial artery (figure 2-10 K).

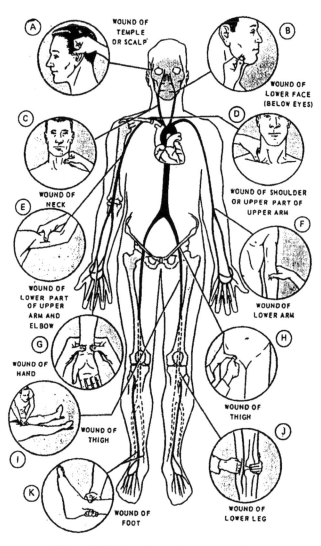

Figure 2-10. Locations of pressure points.

2-14. APPLY A PRESSURE DRESSING

If blood continues to seep from the dressing on a limb after you have applied and secured the field dressing, applied manual pressure, and elevated the wound (if applicable), apply a pressure dressing. The objective of applying a pressure dressing is to stop the bleeding, not to stop all blood circulation below the wound. (Stopping all blood circulation would endanger the body tissue below the pressure dressing.) A pressure dressing is usually not required unless arterial or heavy venous bleeding is involved.

CAUTION: A pressure dressing is applied only to a wound on an arm or leg.

a. **Prepare the Wad.** Make a "wad" by folding material such as a muslin bandage (cravat) from your aid bag, a rag, material torn from clothing, or similar material. Fold the material several times.

b. **Prepare the Bandage.** The wad is secured by a bandage, usually a cravat made from a muslin bandage or similar material. Other materials such as a handkerchief, sock, or strip of cloth torn from a shirt can also be used. Wire and narrow material (such as a shoestring) should not used since they are likely to damage blood vessels and nerve tissue. Cravats can be made from a muslin bandage or from a square of material about three feet on each side in the following manner.

(1)   Fold the square of material along the diagonal (figure 2-11 A) and cut the material in half (figure 2-11 B). You now have two triangular bandages. One triangular bandage is used for the pressure dressing. The remaining triangular bandage can be used to make the tourniquet band, if needed, or used as a sling, swathe, or additional securing bandage.

(2)   Fold the top (apex) of the triangular bandage so it touches the base (cut diagonal) of the triangular bandage (figure 2-11 C). This is a one-fold cravat.

(3)   Fold the material two more times (figures 2-11 D and E).

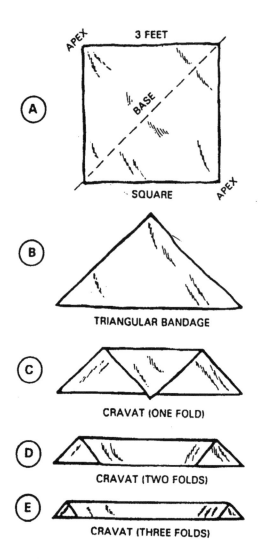

Figure 2-11. Making a cravat from a muslin bandage or similar material.

c. **Position the Wad.** Place the wad of material on top of the field dressing pad directly over the wound (figure 2-12 A).

CAUTION: The pressure dressing is applied on top of the field dressing. The field dressing is <u>not</u> removed or retied. Moving the field dressing would interfere with any clot which had begun to form.

d. **Apply the Bandage.**

(1)   Place the bandage (cravat) over the wad and wrap the bandage tightly around the injured limb (figure 2-12 B).

(2)   Bring the ends of the bandage back over the wound (the ends come from opposite directions), covering the edges of the wad if possible (figure 2-12 C).

e. **Tie the Bandage.** Tie the ends of the bandage in a non-slip knot directly over the wound (figure 2-12 D). The bandage should be tight enough so only the tip of one finger can be inserted under the knot. <u>Do not</u> tie the bandage so tight that it cuts off blood circulation.

f. **Apply Manual Pressure.** Apply additional pressure by pressing firmly with your hand over the pressure dressing. If the casualty is able, have him apply the manual pressure himself.

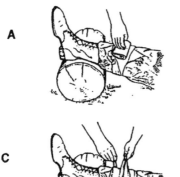
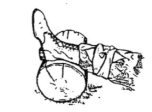

A   B   C   D

Figure 2-12. Applying a pressure dressing.

2-15. CHECK THE CIRCULATION BELOW THE PRESSURE DRESSING

Recheck the casualty's blood circulation and nerve function below the wound. If possible, compare the area below the wound to the same area on the uninjured limb. Use the same procedures given in paragraph 2-8.

2-16. LOOSEN AND RETIE THE PRESSURE DRESSING BANDAGE, IF NEEDED

If the circulation and nerve function below the wound were not impaired before the pressure dressing was applied but are impaired now, the bandage may be too tight. Loosen and retie the bandage; then check the area below the wound again. If circulation and nerve function are not restored, evacuate the casualty as soon as possible.

2-17. EVALUATE THE EFFECTIVENESS OF THE PRESSURE DRESSING

After applying the pressure dressing and manual pressure, check for continued bleeding from the wound.

a. If the wound continues to bleed profusely, apply a tourniquet.

CAUTION: A tourniquet is not used for wounds to the head, neck, or trunk.

NOTE: A tourniquet is not used for a wound on the hand or foot. Bleeding from such injuries can be controlled using a dressing, manual pressure, and elevation.

b. If the bleeding has been controlled, proceed to check the casualty for other injuries. Continue to monitor the pressure dressing. If bleeding begins again, apply manual pressure. Apply a tourniquet, if needed. Also, monitor the casualty for signs of shock (Lesson 7).

2-18. APPLY A TOURNIQUET

A tourniquet is applied only if bleeding from an upper arm, forearm, thigh, or lower leg threatens the casualty's life. Procedures for applying a tourniquet follow.

a. **Select the Tourniquet Site.** Select the area on the limb where you will place the tourniquet band. The site should be two to four inches above the edge of the wound (between the wound and the heart), but not over a joint. If a field dressing has been applied, the tourniquet must be above the edge of the field dressing. If the wound is just below the elbow or knee, select a site above the joint and as close to the joint as possible.

b. **Apply the Combat Application Tourniquet, if Available**. If a Combat Application Tourniquet (CAT) is available, use it.

(1) Remove the CAT from its pouch.

NOTE: The CAT is packaged in its one-handed configuration.

(2) Slide the wounded extremity through the loop of the self-adhering band (figure 2-13) and position the CAT at the tourniquet site (two to four inches <u>above</u> the wound) (figure 2-14).

CAUTION: If the wound is more than four inches <u>below</u> the knee or elbow, initially position the tourniquet band two to four inches above the wound. If a tourniquet applied below the joint does not stop the bleeding, apply a second tourniquet <u>above</u> the joint. <u>Do not</u> remove the first tourniquet until the second tourniquet has been applied.

(3) Pull the free running end of the self-adhering band tight and securely fasten it back on itself (figure 2-15). Do not adhere the band past the windlass clip.

(4) Adhere self-adhering band completely around the limb until the clip is reached (figure 2-16).

(5) Twist the windlass rod until the bright red arterial bleeding has stopped (figure 2-17).

NOTE: Darker bleeding (drainage from the veins) may still continue for a while.

(6) Lock the windlass rod in place with the windlass clip (figure 2-18).

(7) For small extremities, continue to adhere the self-adhering band around the extremity and over the windlass rod (figure 2-19).

(8) Grasp the windlass strap, pull it tight, and adhere it to the Velcro on the windlass clip (figure 2-20).

(9) At this point the tourniquet is secure (figure 2-21).

(a) For added security (and always before moving a casualty) secure the windlass rod with the windlass strap.

(b) For small extremities, also secure the self-adhering band under the windlass strap.

(c) It is recommended that you tape over the entire device and windlass to further secure the tourniquet for transport.

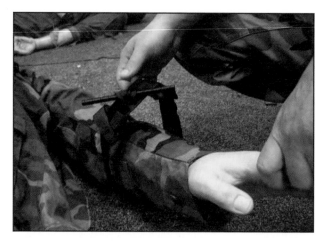

Figure 2-13. Place the wounded extremity through the loop of the self-adhering band.

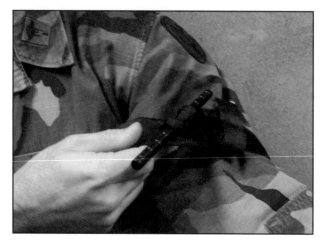

Figure 2-14. Place tourniquet above the injury site.

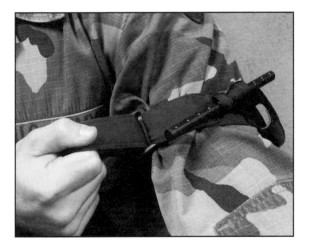

Figure 2-15. Pull the free-running end of the self-adhering band tight and securely fasten it back on itself.

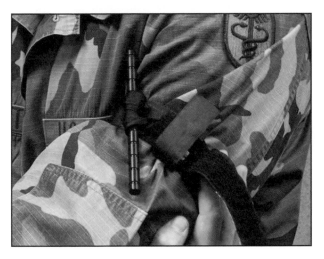

Figure 2-16. Adhere self-adhering band completely around the limb until the clip is reached.

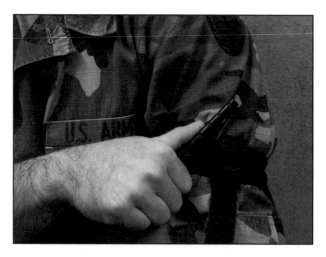

Figure 2-17. Twist the windlass rod until the bleeding has stopped.

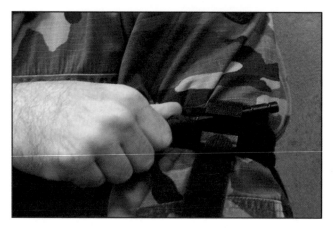

Figure 2-18. Lock the windlass rod in place with the windlass clip.

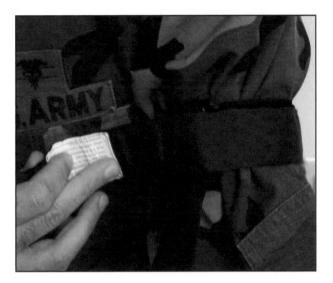

Figure 2-19. For small extremities, continue to adhere the self-adhering band around the extremity and over the windlass rod.

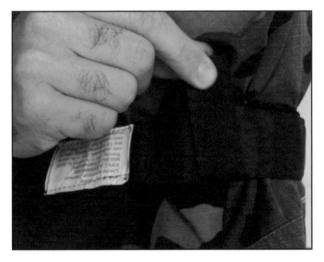

Figure 2-20. Grasp the windlass strap, pull it tight, and adhere it to the Velcro on the windlass clip.

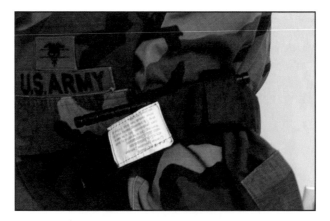

Figure 2-21. CAT tourniquet secured.

(10) The friction adaptor buckle is not necessary for proper CAT application to an arm (figure 2-22). However, it MUST be used when applying to a leg. For this reason it is recommended to prepare all of your CAT in this manner so they will be ready for action (figure 2-23).

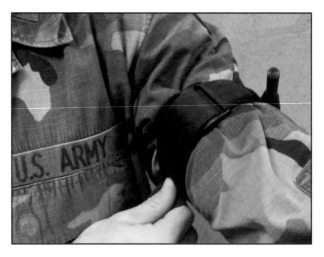

Figure 2-22. Friction adaptor buckle.

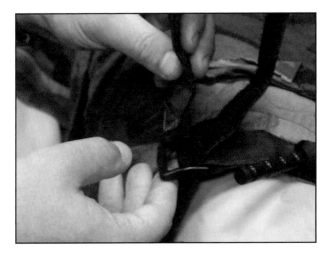

Figure 2-23. Friction buckle being used when applying a CAT to a leg.

    c. **Apply an Improvised Tourniquet, if Needed.** If a CAT is not available, you can apply an improvised tourniquet.

        (1)   A tourniquet can be improvised from a sphygmomanometer if one is available. Place the bladder (blood pressure cuff) around the tourniquet site, tape it completely around to keep the Velcro from popping loose, and inflate the bladder until no pulse is detected below the bladder, and leave the bladder inflated.

        (2)   Procedures for making an improvised tourniquet using a cravat and a rigid object are given in Section III.

        (3)   Many improvised and manufactured tourniquets are available. Some, even those still available through the Army system, may not be effective in stopping all arterial bleeding. The basic cravat and stick tourniquet is still one of the simplest and most effective tourniquets. Research has shown that a tourniquet must have an external windlass or ratcheting device to be effective; so called one-handed tourniquets can not be effectively tightened.

    d. **Check the Effectiveness of the Tourniquet.** Check for a pulse below the tourniquet. If the tourniquet has stopped arterial blood flow, there should be no pulse. Also, the bright red arterial bleeding will have stopped. The darker venous blood may continue to ooze even after the tourniquet has been properly applied. If there is still a pulse below the tourniquet or if arterial bleeding continues, tighten the tourniquet.

2-19. MARK THE CASUALTY

If a tourniquet has been applied, write the letter "T" on the casualty's forehead with a pen, the casualty's blood, mud, or other substance. The information may be written on a piece of tape applied to the casualty's forehead. The "T" alerts medical personnel in the evacuation vehicle and at the medical treatment facility that a tourniquet has been applied. If possible, include the time and date that the tourniquet was applied.

2-20. CONTINUE YOUR SURVEY AND TREATMENT

Continue to examine the casualty. Treat any other life-threatening conditions found during the tactical field care phase, including treating the casualty for hypovolemic shock (Lesson 7).

a. Asses the tourniquet for its appropriateness and effectiveness.

b. Leave the tourniquet exposed. If you cover the casualty to keep him warm, leave the tourniquet in full view so it can be located quickly by other medical personnel.

c. Apply a splint to the injured limb to help prevent additional injury. Be careful to avoid hiding the tourniquet.

d. Periodically reexamine the tourniquet to make sure bleeding has not resumed. If bleeding resumes, tighten the tourniquet.

2-21. DOCUMENT TREATMENT AND EVACUATE THE CASUALTY

a. Initiate a U.S. Field Medical Card (FMC), DD Form 1380. If a tourniquet was applied, enter "Yes" in Block 21. Include the time and date of application. Record any other procedures (field and pressure dressings applied, for example) in Block 20. Instructions for initiating the FMC are given in Subcourse MD0920, Medical Records and Sick Call Procedures.

b. Evacuate the casualty to a medical treatment facility. Use the wire on the FMC to attach the original card to the casualty's clothing before evacuating the casualty. Keep the duplicate (white sheet) in the FMC pad.

Section III. APPLYING AN IMPROVISED TOURNIQUET

2-22. IMPROVISED TOURNIQUETS

Improvised tourniquets are extremely effective and should be readily available. As stated previously, the immediate need for access to a tourniquet is essential to the combat medic. A limited number of manufactured tourniquets may be available. There are many techniques for pre-tying the windlass device to the cravat so that tourniquet application can be faster. The following steps do not address many of these techniques, but they give the good basic technique.

2-23. GATHER MATERIALS FOR MAKING AN IMPROVISED TOURNIQUET

If you do not have a field tourniquet available, you can make an improvised tourniquet. You will need a tourniquet band, a rigid object, and padding materials. Additional securing material may also be needed.

a. **Tourniquet Band.** Obtain a band of strong, pliable, folded material which is at least two inches wide. A cravat made from a folded muslin bandage (figure 2-11) is preferred. A folded handkerchief, a folded strip of clothing, or a belt can also be used as the tourniquet band. Do not use wire, shoestrings, or other narrow materials for the tourniquet band. A wide tourniquet band protects the tissues beneath the tourniquet when it is tightened. Very narrow materials may result in serious damage to the nerves and blood vessels when the tourniquet is tightened.

b. **Rigid Object.** Obtain a rigid object, usually a stick, which is long enough and sturdy enough to tighten the tourniquet band and be secured.

c. **Padding.** Obtain padding material to be placed between the limb and the tourniquet band to protect the skin from being pinched and twisted when the band is tightened. Soft, smooth material should be used for the padding. The casualty's shirt sleeve or trouser leg can be used as padding.

d. **Securing Materials.** Obtain material to be used to secure the rigid object once the tourniquet band has been tightened. If the cravat used as a tourniquet band is long enough, the tails of the cravat can be used to secure the rigid object. Another cravat or strip of cloth similar to the tourniquet band can be used to secure the rigid object.

2-24. APPLY THE TOURNIQUET

a. **Select the Tourniquet Site.** Select a site that is two to four inches above the edge of the wound, but not over a joint or at the edge of the field dressing. If the wound is just below the elbow or knee, select a site above the joint and as close to the joint as possible.

b. **Apply Padding.** Place padding around the limb where the tourniquet will be applied. If the casualty's shirt sleeve or trouser leg is used as padding, smooth the shirt or trouser material and apply the tourniquet band over the clothing.

c. **Apply the Tourniquet Band.** Place the tourniquet band material around the tourniquet site. If possible, wrap the tourniquet band around the limb twice.

d. **Apply the Rigid Object.**

(1) Tie the band with a half knot (figure 2-24 A). This is the same as the first part of tying a shoe.

(2) Place the rigid object on top of the half-knot (figure 2-24 B).

(3) Tie a full knot over the rigid object (figure 2-24 C).

e. **Tighten the Tourniquet.** Twist the rigid object either clockwise or counterclockwise (figure 2-24 D) until the tourniquet is tight enough to stop arterial blood flow beneath the band.

2-25. SECURE THE RIGID OBJECT

Once the tourniquet is tightened, you must secure the rigid object so the tourniquet will not untwist.

a. **Tourniquet Band Tails.** If the remaining tails of the tourniquet band are long enough, use them to secure the rigid object.

(1) Align the rigid object lengthwise (parallel) with the limb.

(2) Wrap one tail of the tourniquet band over and around one end of the rigid object (figure 2-24 E).

(3) Bring that tail down the side of the injured limb.

(4) Wrap the other tail of the tourniquet band over and around the other end of the rigid object.

(5) Bring that tail down the other side of the injured limb.

(6) Bring the tails together and tie them in a nonslip knot under the injured limb (figure 2-24 F).

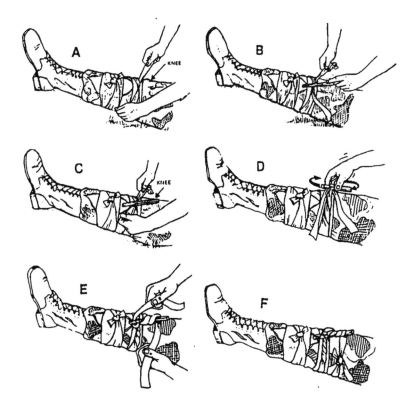

Figure 2-24. Applying an improvised tourniquet to a limb.

    b. **Other Securing Materials.** If the tails are not long enough to secure the rigid object, use a cravat or strip of cloth to secure the object.

        (1)   Wrap the cravat or other piece of material around the limb <u>below</u> the level of the tourniquet band, but near enough to the tourniquet so the rigid object passes over the securing material. Wrap the material around the limb twice, if possible.

NOTE: The rigid object is secured below the tourniquet so the additional securing material will not interfere with blood circulation above the tourniquet.

        (2)   Align the rigid object lengthwise (parallel) with the limb.

(3) Wrap the material around the end of the rigid object so the rigid object is secured. This will prevent the tourniquet from unwinding.

(4) Tie the tails of the material in a non-slip knot.

2-26. CHECK EFFECTIVENESS OF TOURNIQUET

Check for a pulse below the tourniquet. If the tourniquet has stopped arterial blood flow, there should be no pulse. Also, the bright red arterial bleeding will have stopped. If there is still a pulse below the tourniquet or if arterial bleeding continues, tighten the tourniquet.

CAUTION: Leave the tourniquet exposed so it can be located quickly by medical Personnel

2-27. MARK THE CASUALTY AND CONTINUE SURVEY

a. Mark the casualty to indicate that a tourniquet has been applied (paragraph 2-19).

b. Continue to your survey of the casualty (paragraph 2-20).

c. Document treatment on a U.S. Field Medical Card, attach the card to the casualty's clothing, and evacuate the casualty (paragraph 2-21).

Section IV. CONTROLLING BLEEDING FROM AN AMPUTATION

2-28. DETERMINE THE TYPE OF AMPUTATION

An amputation (severing) of a limb is handled somewhat differently than a heavily bleeding wound on a limb. The amputation can be complete or partial. The amputation can be of a limb or a part of the hand or foot.

a. **Complete Amputation**. In a complete amputation, the part of the limb below the amputation site is completely severed (cut off).

b. **Partial Amputation**. In a partial (incomplete) amputation, the portion of the limb below the wound (site of the incomplete amputation) is almost completely severed from the body, but some skin tissue continues to connect the portion of the limb below the wound to the rest of the body.

c. **Amputation of a Limb.** The amputation of a limb exists when the amputation site is on the upper arm, elbow, forearm, wrist, thigh, knee, lower leg, or ankle.

d. **Amputation of Part of a Hand or Foot.** An amputation of a part of the hand exists when the amputation site is below the wrist and does not involve the entire hand. An amputation of a part of the foot exists when the amputation site is below the ankle and does not involve the entire foot.

2-29. APPLY A TOURNIQUET TO AN AMPUTATION OF THE LIMB

A complete or partial amputation of the limb requires the immediate application of a tourniquet. Do not attempt to control bleeding with a field dressing, elevation, manual pressure, and/or pressure dressing before applying a tourniquet. If the amputation is incomplete, do not complete the amputation. There is a possibility the limb may still be saved.

a. **Locate the Tourniquet Site.** Locate a site for the tourniquet that is two to four inches above the wound (amputation site), but which is not over a joint. If the amputation site is just below the elbow or knee, select a site above the joint and as close to the joint as possible.

b. **Apply the Tourniquet.** Apply a Combat Application Tourniquet or an improvised tourniquet. Make sure arterial bleeding below the tourniquet has ceased.

c. **Mark the Casualty.** Mark the casualty's forehead to indicate the application of a tourniquet (paragraph 2-19).

2-30. APPLY A DRESSING TO THE STUMP

Dress and bandage the stump or exposed area of a partial amputation. The dressing will absorb drainage from the wound and help to protect the wound from additional contamination and further injury. This is accomplished during the tactical field care phase as the situation permits. The dressing and bandage should not interfere with or hide the tourniquet. The dressing can be secured with an elastic roller bandage using the recurrent wrap technique described below and in figure 2-25.

NOTE: The tourniquet and the dressing are not shown in figure 2-25. A similar technique can be used to secure a dressing applied to a complete amputation of part of the hand or foot.)

a. Lay the end of the bandage on the limb below the tourniquet and at an angle so one corner (apex) of the bandage is pointing upward.

b. Wrap the bandage completely around the limb; then wrap the bandage around a second time.

c. Turn down the apex (shown as a small triangle in figure 2-25 A) so it lies on top of the second layer of the bandage and wrap the bandage around the limb a third time. The bandage is now anchored.

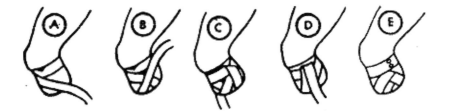

Figure 2-25. Applying a recurrent bandage to a stump.

d. Bring the bandage down diagonally across the front of the limb (figure 2-25 A), over the dressing on the stump to the back of the limb. Hold the bandage in back so it will not slip.

e. Bring the bandage from the back of the limb, over the dressing again, and to the front. Move diagonally up across the front of the limb, forming an "X" pattern with the downward diagonal (figure 2-25 B). Bring the bandage around the limb and to the front.

f. Form the first recurrent (running back to the source). Put your thumb on the top of the bandage to keep it in place, make a fold, bring the bandage down, over the far side of the dressing, and up the back (figure 2-25 C). Hold the dressing in place on the back of the limb with your index finger.

g. Form the second recurrent. Make a fold at the back and bring the bandage down, over the opposite side of the dressing, and up the front (figure 2-25 D).

h. Continue the wrapping procedure. Overlap each layer about one half the width of the previous layer. Continue to hold each succeeding layer securely in place with your thumb and index finger.

i. When the dressing and stump end have been completely covered, reverse the direction of the bandage and make two circular turns to cover the gathered ends you have held with your thumb and index finger. This locks the recurrents in place.

j. Move diagonally down and across the stump from the locking turn, encasing the edges of the recurrents. Then move back diagonally to form another "X" pattern.

k. Overlap the "X" pattern with another circular turn.

l. Secure the end of the bandage (figure 2-25 E). The bandage can be tied, taped, clipped, or pinned.

2-31. CONTINUE YOUR SURVEY AND TREATMENT

Continue your survey and treatment procedures, including treatment for hypovolemic shock. Document treatment on a U.S. Field Medical Card and evacuate the casualty as soon as possible. If the amputate was complete, evacuate the amputated limb with the casualty. There is a possibility that the limb can be reattached.

CAUTION: Make sure the severed body part is kept out of the casualty's sight both before and during evacuation.

Section V. TREATING INTERNAL BLEEDING IN AN EXTREMITY

2-32. IDENTIFY INTERNAL BLEEDING IN AN EXTREMITY

When an artery or vein in an extremity is damaged by a blow or a fractured bone and there is no open wound that will allow the blood to escape, the blood from the damaged blood vessel is trapped in the surrounding tissues. Since the marrow in the center of bones like the femur produces blood cells, a fracture can result in significant internal bleeding even if no major blood vessels are damaged.

a. Internal bleeding into the tissues of the arm or leg can result in hypovolemic shock due to blood loss. Signs and symptoms of hypovolemic shock are given in paragraph 7-2.

b. Other signs of internal bleeding in an extremity include discolored tissue (bruises) and swelling of the injured limb. Swelling can be identified by comparing the circumference of the injured limb to the circumference of the same area on the uninjured limb.

2-33. TREAT INTERNAL BLEEDING IN AN EXTREMITY

Internal bleeding in a limb can be controlled somewhat by applying pressure and a splint to the limb. Initiate an intravenous infusion if signs and symptoms of shock are present and evacuate the casualty. If possible, administer oxygen (high percentage) to the casualty during evacuation.

a. **Pressure.** Apply pressure to the injured limb (paragraphs 2-34 and 2-35).

CAUTION: The pressure should decrease internal bleeding, but should not stop blood circulation. Check circulation in the limb after applying the pressure device.

b. **Immobilization.** Keep the casualty as still as possible. Immobilize (splint) the limb even if it does not appear to be fractured. A splint will apply pressure and help protect the limb from further injury.

2-34. APPLY A SPIRAL WRAP TO AN EXTREMITY

An elastic roller bandage can be applied to a limb to compress the blood vessels and help control bleeding. The bandage also provides support for damaged muscle tissues. A three-inch wide roller bandage is normally used for wrapping the forearm, arm, or calf (lower leg). When wrapping the thigh, a wider bandage (four to six inches wide) is normally used.

a. Expose the limb and check the circulation at a point below the point of injury, such as the wrist or foot.

b. Position the body part to be bandaged in a normal resting position (position of function). The body part should be as clean and dry as possible.

c. Lay the end of the bandage on the bottom of the limb to be wrapped and at an angle so one corner (apex) of the bandage will not be covered when the bandage is brought around the limb (figure 2-26 A).

d. Wrap the bandage completely around the limb twice and past the apex (figure 2-26 B).

e. Fold the apex over the bandage (figure 2-26 C) so that it lies on top of the bandage.

f. Continue wrapping the bandage around the limb a third time, covering the apex with the turn. The bandage is now anchored.

g. Wrap the limb in a spiral manner (figure 2-26 D). On each turn, overlap about one-third of the previous turn. Keep the bandage tight enough to apply pressure to the limb, but not tight enough to impair blood circulation.

h. Continue wrapping until the entire portion of the limb has been wrapped.

i. Secure the wrap with two circular turns at the top of the limb portion being bandaged. Then tape, clip, or tie the end of the bandage in a position that is easy to reach (figure 2-26 E).

j. Check circulation below the bandage. If blood circulation was not impaired before the bandage was applied but is now impaired, loosen the bandage and apply the bandage again.

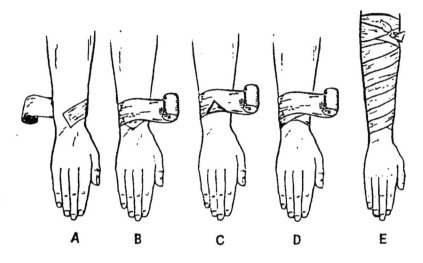

Figure 2-26. Applying a spiral bandage to a forearm.

2-35. APPLY A SPIRAL REVERSE WRAP TO AN EXTREMITY

Although the spiral wrap is normally used to apply pressure to a limb, the spiral reverse wrap can also be used. The spiral reverse wrap is especially useful when applying pressure to the calf (lower leg) since it follows the contours of the limb more closely than does the spiral wrap.

a. Expose the limb and check the circulation at a point below the injury, such as the foot.

b. Lay the end of the bandage on the bottom of the limb to be wrapped and at an angle so one corner (apex) of the bandage will not be covered when the bandage is brought around the limb.

NOTE: In figure 2-26, the apex points down toward the hand. In figure 2-27, the apex points up away from the foot. Either method is acceptable.

c. Wrap the bandage completely around the limb twice and past the starting point.

d. Fold the apex (figure 2-27 A) so it lies on top of the bandage.

e. Continue wrapping the bandage around the limb a third time, bringing the bandage over and covering the apex. The bandage is now anchored.

f. Wrap the limb in a spiral manner (figure 2-27 B) for a couple of turns.

g. Make a spiral reverse turn (figure 2-27 C).

(1) Place your thumb on the upper edge of the bandage and hold firmly.

(2) Turn the bandage down over the thumb and toward the lower edge of the previous turn.

(3) Cover about half of the previous lap and continue the turn.

h. Continue making spiral reverse turns until the entire portion of the limb has been wrapped. Keep the bandage tight enough to apply pressure to the limb, but not tight enough to impair blood circulation.

i. Secure the wrap with two circular turns at the top of the limb portion being bandaged. Then tape, clip, or tie the end of the bandage in a position that is easy to reach (figure 2-27 D).

j. Check circulation below the bandage. If blood circulation was not impaired before the bandage was applied but has become impaired, loosen the bandage and apply the bandage again.

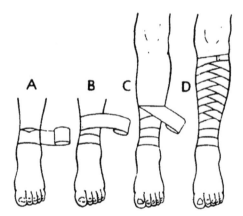

Figure 2-27. Applying a reverse spiral bandage to a lower leg.

Continue with Exercises

EXERCISES, LESSON 2

INSTRUCTIONS: Answer the following exercises by marking the lettered response that best answers the question or best completes the sentence or by writing the answer in the space provided.

After you have answered all of the exercises, turn to "Solutions to Exercises" at the end of the lesson and check your answers. For each exercise answered incorrectly, reread the lesson material referenced with the solution.

1. The pad of material placed on the wound to absorb the blood is called

   the _____; the material used to keep the pad of material from

   slipping off the wound is the _____.

2. A casualty has a deep cut on his leg. Bright red blood is being expelled from the wound in spurts. This casualty probably has:

   a. A severed artery.

   b. A severed capillary.

   c. A severed vein.

   d. Internal bleeding.

3. While surveying your casualty under enemy fire, you discover the casualty is bleeding heavily from a wound in the thigh. The blood appears bluish-red and is flowing from the wound at a steady rate. You should:

   a. Take immediate measures to control the bleeding.

   b. Wait until you are in the tactical field care phase to treat the bleeding.

   c. Wait until you are in the combat casualty evacuation care phase to treat the bleeding.

4. Why should you push away any loose clothing near a casualty's open wound before applying a field dressing?

   a. To allow the wound to get air.

   b. To provide a sterile work area.

   c. To apply ointment to the wound.

   d. To see the extent of the wound.

5. A casualty is bleeding from a wound in the leg. Part of the trouser material is stuck to the wound. You should:

   a. Gently pull the stuck material from the wound.

   b. Cut around the stuck material so it will be free from the rest of the trouser material. The stuck material should not be removed from the wound.

6. Under what conditions should the tourniquet be removed?

   a. NEVER, this will allow the casualty to continue bleeding.

   b. Periodically, to return circulation to the limb

   c. Under proper conditions when time is on your side.

7. When applying a field dressing to a bleeding wound on the arm, the tails should be tied in a non-slip knot:

   a. Directly over the center of the wound.

   b. At the edge of the dressing.

   c. On the other side of the arm (away from the wound).

   d. Wherever the tails happen to cross.

8. After applying a field dressing to a bleeding wound on the casualty's

forearm, you should _____ the arm if the arm is not _____.

9. When elevating a leg with a bleeding wound which has been dressed, you should:

a. Elevate the leg above the level of the casualty's heart by placing it on a pack.

b. Elevate the leg as high as possible.

10. When applying digital pressure to help control bleeding from a wound on an extremity, you should apply pressure to the artery at a point:

a. Above the wound.

b. Below the wound.

11. Which of the following is applied with the intent of stopping all arterial blood flow to the wound?

a. Field dressing.

b. Elevation of the limb.

c. Pressure dressing.

d. None of the above.

12. A pressure dressing is usually:

a. Another field dressing applied on top of the first field dressing.

b. Another field dressing applied 2 to 4 inches above the first field dressing.

c. Folded material applied on top of the field dressing and secured by a cravat.

13. When applying a pressure dressing, the tails should be tied:

    a. Directly over the wound.

    b. Over the outer edge of the dressing.

    c. On the other side of the limb (away from the wound).

    d. Wherever the tails happen to cross.

14. The portion of the limb below the pressure dressing has become cool to

    the touch and the nail beds on the limb are turning bluish. The pressure

    dressing should be _____ and _____.

    If the condition does not improve _____ the casualty.

15. Normally, a tourniquet should be applied _____ to _____ inches
    above (closer to the heart than) the wound.

16. If the amputation site is about one inch below the elbow joint, the tourniquet is
    applied:

    a. Between the wound and the elbow.

    b. Directly over the elbow.

    c. Slightly above the elbow.

    d. Four to six inches above the elbow.

17. You and the casualty are not in danger from enemy fire. In which of the following situations would you apply a tourniquet without first trying to control the bleeding with a pressure dressing?

    a. Severe bleeding from a wound on the leg.

    b. Severe bleeding from a wound on the forearm.

    c. Amputation of the arm near the elbow.

    d. Amputation of two or more toes.

18. Which of the following is preferred for an improvised tourniquet band?

    a. A wire that is 36 inches long.

    b. A bootlace.

    c. A rubber band.

    d. A muslin bandage folded into a cravat about three inches wide.

19. Should padding be placed between the tourniquet band and the casualty's limb?

    a. Yes.

    b. No.

20. Which one of the following statements gives a proper rule for tightening a tourniquet?

    a. A tourniquet should be loose enough so that you can slip two fingers under the tourniquet band.

    b. A tourniquet should be loose enough so that you can slip the tip of one finger under the tourniquet band.

    c. A tourniquet is to be tightened until the bright red bleeding has stopped; darker blood oozing from the wound can be ignored.

    d. A tourniquet is to be tightened until both the bright red bleeding and the darker venous bleeding have stopped completely.

21. Once you have tightened the tourniquet band of an improvised tourniquet, you must:

    a. Apply a field dressing over the rigid object.

    b. Check the casualty's carotid pulse.

    c. Remove the rigid object and tie the tails in a non-slip knot.

    d. Secure the rigid object so the tourniquet will not unwind.

22. Once the tourniquet has been applied, should it be covered with a blanket, poncho, or similar material?

    a. Yes.

    b. No.

23. The casualty's forearm arm has suffered a complete amputated slightly above the wrist. You have applied a tourniquet. How is the stump treated?

    a. The stump is dressed and bandaged.

    b. The stump is left exposed to facilitate drainage.

24. After you have applied a tourniquet, you should write the

    letter _____ and the _____ the tourniquet was applied on

    the casualty's _____.

25. A casualty has internal bleeding in a limb. Which of the following should you do to help to control the bleeding?

    a. Apply a tourniquet to the limb.

    b. Apply pressure to the limb using elastic roller bandages to form a spiral wrap.

Check Your Answers on Next Page

SOLUTIONS TO EXERCISES, LESSON 2

1. Dressing, bandage.   (paras 2-4b, c)

2. a   (para 2-2a(1))

3. a   (paras 2-2a(2), 2-5)

4. d   (para 2-7)

5. b   (para 2-7h)

6. c   (para 2-5a)

7. b   (para 2-9d(4))

8. Elevate, fractured (or broken).   (para 2-11)

9. a   (para 2-11b)

10. a   (para 2-13)

11. d   (paras 2-10, 2-11, 2-16)

12. c   (para 2-14)

13. a   (para 2-14e)

14. Loosened, retied; evacuate.   (para 2-16)

15. Two, four.   (para 2-18a)

16. c   (para 2-18a)

17. c   (para 2-29)

18. d   (para 2-23a)

19. a   (para 2-23c)

20. c   (paras 2-18f, f Note, 2-24e20d)

21. d   (para 2-25)

22. b   (para 2-20b)

23. a   (para 2-30)

24. T; time and date; forehead.   (para 2-19)

25. b   (paras 2-33a, 2-34)

End of Lesson 2

LESSON 3	Treating Chest Injuries.
TEXT ASSIGNMENT	Paragraphs 3-1 through 3-25.
LESSON OBJECTIVES	When you have completed this lesson, you should be able to:

3-1. Identify the signs and symptoms of an open chest wound.

3-2. Identify the procedures for treating a casualty with an open chest wound.

3-3. Identify the signs and symptoms of a closed chest injury.

3-4. Identify the procedures for treating a casualty with a closed chest injury.

SUGGESTION   Work the lesson exercises at the end of this lesson before beginning the next lesson. These exercises will help you accomplish the lesson objectives.

LESSON 3

TREATING CHEST INJURIES

Section I. GENERAL

3-1. THORACIC CAVITY

The chest is also called the thorax. The thoracic (chest) cavity is the body cavity located between the neck and the diaphragm. It is surrounded by the rib cage (figure 3-1). The thoracic cavity contains the lungs, the heart, and many major blood vessels. Any injury to the chest can be serious. A penetrating object, for example, can puncture a lung, an artery or vein, or the heart itself.

3-2. RIB CAGE

The rib cage includes the ribs, the 12 thoracic vertebrae (spine), and sternum (breastbone). The ribs are connected to the vertebrae in back and all but four ribs (the lowest two pairs) are connected to the sternum in front by cartilage. The small spear-like structure at the bottom of the sternum is the xiphoid process. Damage to the rib cage can interfere with breathing since the movement of the rib cage assists in inhalation and exhalation. (See Subcourse MD0532, Cardiopulmonary Resuscitation, for additional information on the mechanics of respiration.)

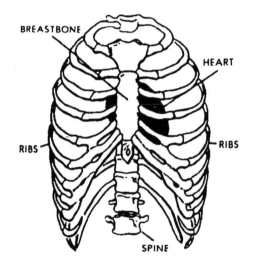

Figure 3-1. Rib cage (showing location of heart).

3-3. ORGANS AND CAVITIES WITHIN THE CHEST

a. **Lungs.** The body has two lungs. Each lung is enclosed in a pleural cavity, which is an airtight area within the chest. Each pleural cavity is separate and independent of the other pleural cavity. If an object punctures the chest wall and allows air to enter one pleural cavity, the lung within that cavity begins to collapse (not expand fully). The other lung, however, will not collapse. Any degree of collapse, though, interferes with the ability to inhale a sufficient amount of air. A buildup of pressure from air or blood around the collapsed lung can also cause compression of the heart and the other lung.

b. **Heart.** The heart is located in the pericardial cavity. The pericardial cavity is located between the lungs in a space called the mediastinum. In addition to the heart, the mediastinum contains the lower part of the trachea, part of the esophagus, large blood vessels, and the thymus.

Section II. TREATING OPEN CHEST WOUNDS

3-4. IDENTIFY A CASUALTY WITH AN OPEN CHEST WOUND

An open chest wound is a wound in which the skin and the chest wall are penetrated. An open chest wound can be caused by a bullet, knife blade, shrapnel, or other object. Some of the signs and symptoms of an open chest wound are given below.

a. Sucking or hissing sounds coming from chest wound. When a casualty with an open chest wound inhales, air goes in the wound. When he exhales, air escapes from the wound. This airflow sometimes causes a "sucking" or "hissing" sound. Because of this distinct sound, an open chest wound is often called a "sucking chest wound."

b. Difficulty in breathing (dyspnea).

c. Visible puncture wound in the chest (front or back). If you are not sure if a wound has penetrated the chest wall completely, treat the wound as though it were an open chest wound.

d. Impaled object protruding from the chest.

e. Frothy blood or air bubbles in the blood around the wound site.

f. Bright red or frothy blood being coughed up.

g. Sputum containing blood.

h. Chest not rising normally during inhalation.

i. Pain in the shoulder or chest area. The pain usually increases with breathing]

j. Bluish tint (cyanosis) of the lips, inside of the mouth, the fingertips, or nail beds. This color change is caused by the decreased amount of oxygen in the blood.

3-5. EXPOSE THE OPEN CHEST WOUND

NOTE: These treatments are conducted during the tactical field care phase.

Expose the area around the open chest wound by removing, unfastening, cutting, or tearing the clothing covering the wound. Do not disrupt the wound any more than is necessary. Do not try to clean the wound or remove debris from the wound.

a. **Chemical Environment.** If you are in a chemical environment, make sure the casualty remains masked. Do not remove the casualty's protective clothing. Cut the casualty's protective clothing (if necessary) to expose the wound, apply sealing material to the wound, apply a dressing (tails go on outside the protective clothing), and repair the protective clothing as quickly as possible. Evacuate the casualty as soon as possible.

b. **Stuck Material.** If clothing or other material is stuck to the wound area, do not remove the stuck material since removing it might cause additional damage to the wound. Cut around the material so the seal and dressing can be applied on top of the stuck material.

c. **Protruding Object.** If an impaled object is protruding from the wound, do not remove the object.

3-6. CHECK FOR OTHER OPEN CHEST WOUNDS

Check for an exit wound. Look for a pool of blood under the casualty's back. Carefully palpate and visually examine the casualty's chest, back, and axillary (armpits) for other open chest wounds. Remove clothing, as needed, to expose other wounds if you are not in a chemical environment. If there is more than one open chest wound, treat the most serious (largest or heaviest bleeding) wound first. Then seal and dress the other open chest wounds. Any wound from the chin to the umbilicus (navel) has the potential to enter the chest cavity and requires the use of an occlusive dressing.

3-7. SEAL THE OPEN CHEST WOUND

One of the objectives in treating an open chest wound is to keep air from entering the chest cavity through the wound. Stopping air from entering the wound helps to keep the lung from collapsing or, at least, slows down the collapse. Since air can pass through a field dressing, airtight sealing material must be placed between the wound and the dressing to keep air from entering the wound.

a. **Manufactured Devices.** Use a manufactured chest seal device if one is available.

(1)   Obtain an Asherman chest seal (figure 3-2) or other appropriate manufactured chest seal device from your aid bag.

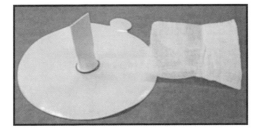

Figure 3-2. The Asherman chest seal.

(2)   Use the included gauze to dry the area surrounding the wound as well as possible to increase adhesion with the dressing.

(3)   If available apply tincture of benzoin around the wound area to increase adhesion of the dressing.

(4)   If the patient has excessive chest hair, the area may need to be shaved to allow proper adhesion of the dressing.

(5)   Remove the backing and expose the adhesive dressing.

(6)   Tell the casualty to exhale and hold his breath. This forces some of the trapped air out of the chest cavity. The more air forced out of the chest cavity before the wound is dressed, the better the casualty will be able to breathe.

NOTE: If the casualty is unconscious or cannot hold his breath, place the adhesive dressing over the wound after his chest falls but before it rises again.

(7)   Apply the adhesive dressing (5.5 inches in diameter) over the wound so that it adheres to the casualty's chest and the one-way valve is over the penetrating wound. The one-way valve lets air and blood escape while preventing their re-entry. The clear pad design allows you to visually inspect the wound.

b. **Improvised Occlusive Dressing**. If you do not have a manufactured seal available, you can improvise a seal using airtight material, such as the plastic envelope from a field dressing or a petroleum gauze packet. The following steps give procedures for sealing an open chest wound using a plastic envelope.

(1)   Obtain a field dressing package. If the casualty is carrying a field dressing, use his dressing. Otherwise, obtain a field dressing from your aid bag.

(2)   Open the plastic dressing envelope.

(a)   Remove the bandage scissors from your aid bag.

(b)   Cut one of the short ends of the plastic envelope and remove the inner packet (dressing wrapped in paper). Cut the envelope so as little as possible is cut off the main part of the envelope. Drop or place the inner packet where it will not become contaminated. You may place the packet on the casualty's abdomen, for example.

(c)   Cut the other short end of the plastic envelope and one of the long sides. You now have a rectangular piece of airtight plastic which can be used to seal the open chest wound.

CAUTION: Avoid touching the inside surface of the plastic envelope. The inner surface will be applied directly to the wound and should be kept as free from contamination as possible.

(3)   Have the casualty exhale.

(a)   If the casualty is conscious, tell him to exhale and hold his breath. This forces some of the trapped air out of the chest cavity. The more air forced out of the chest cavity before the wound is dressed, the better the casualty will be able to breathe.

(b)   If the casualty is unconscious or cannot hold his breath, place the plastic envelope over the wound after his chest falls but before it rises again.

(4) Place sealing material over the wound.

(a) Place the inside surface of the plastic envelope (the side without printing) directly on the chest wound to seal the wound (figure 3-3).

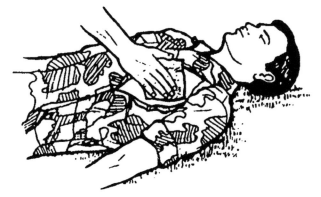

Figure 3-3. Applying sealing material to an open chest wound.

(b) Check the plastic envelope to make sure it extends two inches or more beyond the edges of the wound in all directions. If the envelope does not have a two-inch margin, it may not form an airtight seal and may even be sucked into the wound.

(c) If the envelope is not large enough or is torn, use foil, material cut from a poncho, cellophane, a plastic MRE (meal ready-to-eat) package, or similar airtight material to form the seal.

CAUTION: If an impaled object is protruding from the chest wound, place airtight material around the object to form as airtight a seal as possible.

(5) Tape sealing material in place. Use the tape from your aid bag to tape down all four edges of the plastic envelope.   When the casualty inhales, the plastic is sucked against the wound and air cannot enter the wound.

CAUTION: If the sealing material is not taped down, it must be held in place until the dressing is applied. If the casualty is able, he can hold the sealing material in place. Otherwise, you must keep the sealing material in place while you prepare to dress the wound.

NOTE: Figure 3-4 shows a petroleum gauze packet being used to seal a sucking chest wound.

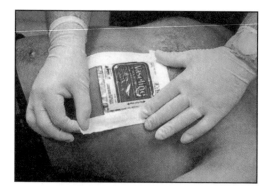

Figure 3-4. Petroleum gauze improvised occlusive dressing.

3-8. DRESS THE OPEN CHEST WOUND

Apply a dressing to secure and protect the seal and to absorb secretions. Secure the dressing with a bandage. The following steps are for applying a field dressing to an improvised occlusive dressing.

a. **Apply the Field Dressing.**

(1) Pick up the packet containing the dressing.

(2) Grasp the packet with both hands and twist until the paper wrapper breaks.

(3) Remove the dressing from the wrapper and discard the wrapper. Avoid touching the white, sterile dressing pad and keep the pad as free from contamination as possible.

(4) Grasp the folded tails of the dressing with both hands, hold the dressing above the wound with the sterile pad toward the wound, and pull the tails so the dressing opens and flattens.

(5) Place the sterile dressing pad on top of the sealing material.

CAUTION: If an impaled object is protruding from the chest wound, apply a bulky dressing to the wound without covering or moving the object. Then stabilize the object by placing bulky dressings made from the cleanest material available around the protruding object.

b. **Secure the Dressing.** Secure the dressing using the attached bandages. The bandages must be tight enough to ensure the dressing will not slip, but not tight enough to interfere with the casualty's breathing. If the casualty is able, have him hold the dressing in place while you secure it. If he cannot help, hold the dressing in place while securing it (figure 3-5 A).

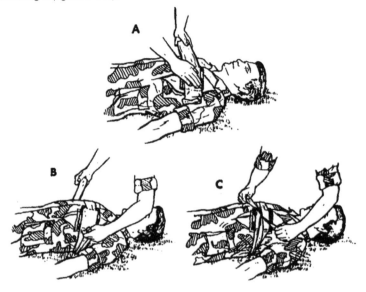

Figure 3-5. Applying a field dressing to an open chest wound.

(1)　Grasp one tail, slide it under the casualty, bring it up the other side of the casualty, and bring it back over the dressing.

(2)　Wrap the other tail around the casualty in the opposite direction (figure 3-5 B) and bring it back over the dressing.

(3)　Tell the casualty to exhale and hold his breath. If the casualty is unconscious or cannot hold his breath, tie the knot after his chest falls and before the chest rises again.

(4)　Tighten the tails and tie them with a non-slip knot over the center of the dressing (figure 3-5 C). Tying the knot over the middle of the dressing directly over the wound will provide additional pressure to the wound and will help to ensure a good seal against the influx of air.

CAUTION: If an object is protruding from the wound, apply additional bandages to hold the bulky dressings in place. <u>Do not</u> wrap the bandages around the protruding object. Tie the bandages in a nonslip knot beside the object, not on it.

    (5) Have the casualty resume normal breathing.

    c. **Apply Additional Padding, If Needed.** Additional pressure and stability can be achieved by placing padding material or other dressings over the field dressing and securing the material with bandages, an elastic roller bandage, or the casualty's belt. Make sure the padding and securing materials do not interfere with the casualty's breathing.

3-9. DRESS AND SEAL THE OTHER OPEN CHEST WOUNDS, IF ANY

    If there is more than one open chest wound, seal and dress the other wound(s) using the same procedures. If improvised dressings and bandages are needed, make dressings from the cleanest material available and use material torn from a shirt or other material as bandages.

3-10. COMPLETE SURVEY

    After the open chest wounds have been sealed and dressed, continue your evaluation and administer any other needed care, including procedures to control shock.

3-11. POSITION THE CASUALTY

    Position the casualty in the position of comfort if he is conscious. Most personnel will request to sit up. This acceptable if the tactical situation permits. If the casualty is unconscious and can not protect his own airway, place the casualty in the recovery position.

    a. **On Side.** Positioning the casualty on his side aids in maintaining an open airway and helps fluids to drain from the casualty's mouth. There is controversy over which side to lay the casualty on. Your local protocols should dictate this. Figure 3-6 shows a casualty in the recovery position lying on his injured side. Pressure from contact with the ground acts like a splint and helps to reduce pain. Since the pressure is on the casualty's injured side, the other (uninjured) lung is not restricted and can inflate fully during inhalation.

    b. **Sitting Up.** The casualty may wish to sit up. If he can breathe easier when sitting up than lying on his injured side, allow him to sit up with his back against a tree, wall, or other stable support. If the casualty becomes tired, position him in the recovery position.

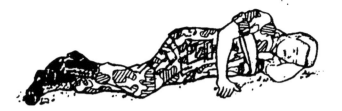

Figure 3-6. Casualty with a dressed open chest wound positioned on his injured side.

3-12. MONITOR THE CASUALTY

Once your surveys are completed and the casualty has been treated, initiate a U.S. Field Medical Card and monitor the casualty. Check the casualty's breathing and his vital signs. Administer oxygen if available. Observe for signs of tension pneumothorax. Evacuate the casualty as soon as possible.

3-13. TREAT TENSION PNEUMOTHORAX, IF NEEDED

a. Tension pneumothorax is a condition in which air continues to accumulate in the pleural cavity and increases pressure on the injured lung. Signs of tension pneumothorax include increased difficulty in breathing, shortness of breath, cyanosis, and the trachea moving from its normal position toward the uninjured side of the chest.

b. If signs of tension pneumothorax are present, perform a chest needle decompression. On the battlefield, unilateral penetrating chest trauma with progressive increases in difficulty breathing is an indication to perform chest needle decompression since other methods of assessment may be unavailable or impossible to assess.

c. If tension pneumothorax is present, perform a chest needle decompression using the following steps. The decompression is performed on the injured side of the chest (side of open chest wound). It allows the air that has become trapped within the chest to escape.

(1) Obtain a 14 gauge needle from the casualty's first aid kit or from your aid bag. The needle should be two to three and a fourth inches in length to ensure it penetrates deep enough into the chest cavity. A catheter covers most of the needle, but does not cover the needle point

(2) Locate the second intercostal space (between second and third rib) on the mid-clavicular line (figure 3-7) on the injured side of the chest.

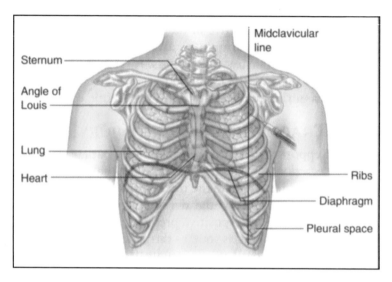

Figure 3-7. Needle position on the mid-clavicular line above the third rib.

     (3)   Prepare the area with anti-microbial scrub if time permits.

     (4)   Insert the needle point at a 90 degree angle over the top of the third rib into the second intercostal space (figure 3-8). Stop advancing the needle once a hiss of air is heard. You should feel a "pop" as the needle enters the chest cavity or you aspirate air (if using a syringe/needle combination).

NOTE: Over insertion of the needle can cause damage to underlying lung tissue or other vital organs. Care must be taken not to over insert the needle.

     (5)   Hold the catheter in place and remove the needle. Safely dispose of the needle.

     (6)   Tape the catheter in place and monitor the casualty. The catheter can be left in place as needed and flushed with saline every two hours to ensure patency. If the mission dictates, it may be advisable to remove the catheter and then monitor the patient closely for signs of building tension and then "re-needle" the chest if necessary. REMEMBER: Once the patient develops a tension pnuemothorax, he will continue to develop tension until the patient receives a chest tube. The patient must be monitored closely.

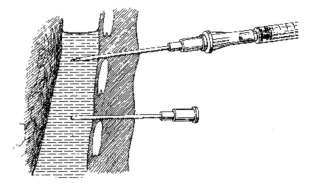

Figure 3-8. Examples of proper needle insertion.

d. If the ability to perform a needle decompression is not available loosen the bandages and lift the sealing material so the trapped air escapes from the pleural cavity. Then apply the sealing material to the wound again and tie the bandages.

Section III. TREATING CLOSED CHEST INJURIES

3-14. IDENTIFY A CASUALTY WITH A CLOSED CHEST INJURY

In a closed chest injury, the chest is injured but there is no break in the skin. A closed chest injury can be caused by a blow to the chest by a blunt instrument, a fall, a cave-in, or a vehicle accident. The following are signs and symptoms of a closed chest injury.

a. Pain in the chest area. The pain may be due to injury to the rib cage and muscles (pain indicates the site of the injury) or to pleurisy (inflammation within the chest cavity). The pain usually increases when the casualty breathes.

b. Labored breathing or difficulty in breathing (dyspnea).

c. Diminished breathing sounds or absence of such sounds.

d. Rapid and weak pulse with low blood pressure.

e. Cyanosis (bluish tint) usually seen first in the lips, nail beds, or inside the mouth.

f. Failure of one or both sides of the chest to expand normally when the casualty inhales.

g. Paradoxical breathing. Paradoxical breathing, an indication of a flail chest, occurs when part of the chest moves in when the casualty inhales and out when the casualty exhales--the opposite of normal motion.

h. Coughing up blood (hemoptysis) or bloody sputum.

i. Enlarged neck veins.

j. Bulging tissue between the ribs or above the clavicles (collarbones). This sign is an indication of tension pneumothorax or hemothorax.

k. Tracheal deviation (a shift of the trachea from its normal midline toward the unaffected side of the casualty's body). The shift is caused by the buildup of pressure on the injured side due to tension pneumothorax. Tracheal deviation is a very late sign.

l. Mediastinal shift (movement of the mediastinum--heart, great blood vessels, trachea, and esophagus--from its normal position toward the unaffected side of the body). Mediastinal shift is caused by the buildup of pressure due to tension pneumothorax or hemothorax.

CAUTION: Mediastinal shift indicates a life-threatening condition (compression of the heart and blood vessels). The pressure must be relieved as soon as possible by trained medical personnel.

3-15. CHECK FOR A FRACTURED RIB

A simple fracture of a rib is usually caused by a direct blow to the chest or by compression of the chest. The casualty usually has local pain at the site of the fracture and the pain is usually aggravated when he breathes or moves. There may be a bruise or swelling at the fracture site. The most common fracture sites are the fifth to the tenth pair of ribs. The upper pairs of ribs are protected by the bones of the shoulders. The lower (eleventh and twelfth) pairs of ribs are not attached to the sternum and have greater flexibility.

3-16. TREAT A CASUALTY WITH A FRACTURED RIB

a. **Immobilize the Fracture.** Make the casualty comfortable and keep him as still as possible. Apply a sling and swathe to the arm on the injured side (figure 3-9). The sling and swathe help to immobilize the injured side as much as possible. There is a danger the rib may be broken in two places. If so, a rib segment is free of the sternum and spine and the segment may "float." The sharp end of the rib segment could puncture the lung or damage the heart or major blood vessels. Subcourse MD0533, Treating Fractures in the Field, describes the procedures for applying slings and swathes.

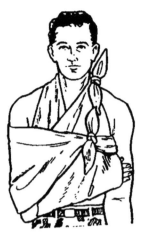

Figure 3-9. Sling and swathe applied to a casualty with a fractured rib.

CAUTION: <u>Do not</u> tape, strap, or bind the chest since these actions could interfere with the casualty's breathing. The swathe should not be tight enough to compress the casualty's chest.

b. **Monitor and Evacuate Casualty.** Monitor the casualty's breathing. Encourage the casualty to take deep breaths to inflate his lungs. If the casualty has difficulty breathing, establish and maintain an open airway. Administer oxygen if it is needed and is available. Observe the casualty for signs and symptoms of tension pneumothorax and hemothorax. Evacuate the casualty when possible.

3-17. CHECK FOR A FLAIL CHEST

A flail chest results when three or more ribs are broken in two or more places, allowing rib segments to "float" (figure 3-10). The sternum may also be fractured. Floating rib segments may damage a lung, major blood vessels, or the heart. Lung tissue lying under the flail segment is usually damaged, resulting in internal bleeding and swelling which interferes with respiratory function.

a. The floating rib segments do not follow the normal chest movements. Their movement is paradoxical (opposite normal) in that the floating rib segments move in when the casualty inhales and out when the casualty exhales.

b. Other indications of a flail chest include a lack of lung expansion resulting in loss of effective lung volume. The casualty usually tries to breathe deeply to offset the decrease in lung efficiency. Severe hypoxia and cyanosis can occur quickly in spite of the casualty's efforts.

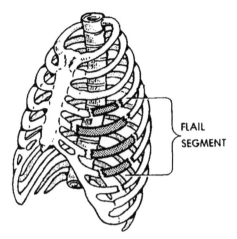

FLAIL
SEGMENT

Figure 3-10. Example of a flail chest.

3-18. TREAT A CASUALTY WITH A FLAIL CHEST

a. **Immobilize the Fracture.** Tape a pillow, folded blanket, field jacket, or poncho in place over the fractures to act as a splint. Have the casualty lie on his injured side. The ground acts like a splint to help restrict movement. This position also helps to reduce pain.

CAUTION: <u>Do not</u> wrap the casualty's chest with tape since the pressure could interfere with the casualty's respirations.

b. **Monitor and Evacuate Casualty.** Monitor the casualty's breathing. If the casualty has difficulty breathing, establish and maintain an open airway. Assist with the casualty's respirations (mouth-to-mouth resuscitation), if needed. Administer oxygen if it is available. Observe the casualty for signs and symptoms of tension pneumothorax and hemothorax. Evacuate the casualty as soon as possible.

3-19. CHECK FOR A COMPRESSION INJURY

A compression injury is caused by the sudden and severe circumferential compression of the rib cage. It can be caused by a motor vehicle accident, cave-in, fall, or other source of severe blunt chest injury. Signs and symptoms of a compression injury include the following.

a. Multiple rib fractures, which may included a flail chest.

b. A feeling of increased pressure within the chest.

c. Distended neck veins.

d. Bulging eyes.

e. Pulmonary contusion.

f. Severe respiratory distress.

g. Cyanosis.

3-20. TREAT A CASUALTY WITH A COMPRESSION INJURY

Establish and maintain an open airway. Assist with the casualty's respirations, if needed. Administer oxygen if it is available. Observe the casualty for signs and symptoms of tension pneumothorax and hemothorax. Evacuate the casualty as soon as possible.

3-21. CHECK FOR A BACK INJURY

Check for injury to the back of the chest. The most important is injury to the spine. Other injuries include lacerations, muscle strain, and fractures of bones associated with the chest (such as the scapula).

3-22. TREAT A CASUALTY WITH A BACK INJURY

Maintain an open airway and assist with respirations, if needed. Keep the casualty as still as possible if a spinal injury is suspected. Procedures for treating a suspected injury to the spine are covered in Subcourse MD0533, Treating Fractures in the Field.

3-23. CHECK FOR TENSION PNEUMOTHORAX AND HEMOTHORAX

a. **Tension Pneumothorax.** Tension pneumothorax is a condition in which air enters the pleural cavity outside the lung and becomes trapped. As more and more air becomes trapped, the increased pressure causes the lung in the affected pleural cavity to collapse. Tension pneumothorax can be caused by an open chest wound (Section II), but it can also result from a closed chest injury. Figure 3-11 shows tension pneumothorax resulting from air that has escaped from a lung injured by floating rib segments. Tension pneumothorax can also result from damage to the bronchi (air tubes) leading to the lungs. Air in the pleural cavity that results from disease rather than trauma to the lung is referred to as spontaneous pneumothorax. Complete collapse of the lung may be followed by tracheal deviation and mediastinal shift. Signs of tension pneumothorax include increased difficulty in breathing, shortness of breath, absent or diminished breath sounds on the effected side, subcutaneous emphysema, distended neck veins, bulging chest tissues, weak pulse, and cyanosis.

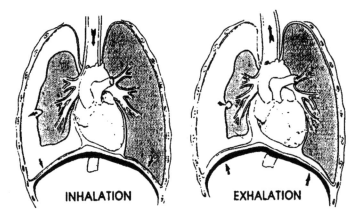

INHALATION   EXHALATION

Figure 3-11. Tension pneumothorax resulting from a closed chest injury.

b. **Hemothorax.** Hemothorax is a condition in which blood enters the pleural cavity outside the lung and becomes trapped. As more and more blood becomes trapped, the increased pressure causes the lung in the affected pleural cavity to collapse (figure 3-12). Hemothorax can be caused by any chest injury. It can result from lacerated blood vessels in the chest wall, lacerated major blood vessels within the chest, or laceration of the lung. Signs and symptoms of tension pneumothorax also apply to hemothorax. In addition, hemothorax may result in hypovolemic shock. Tension pneumothorax and hemothorax may be present together. A hemothorax is more likely to cause significant hypovolemia before tension could be built up. The left and right lung spaces and the mediastinum can hold more than three liters of fluid (over half of the circulating blood volume).

NOTE: Figures 3-11 and 3-12 do not show a significant trachea deviation or mediastinal shift. As the pressure increases and the injured (right) lung collapses, the trachea and heart will be pushed more and more toward the casualty's uninjured (left) side. The shift will compress the heart and the uninjured (left) lung.

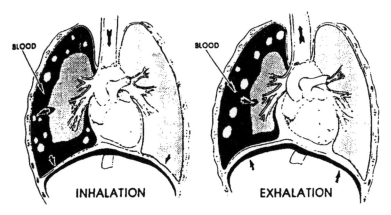

INHALATION   EXHALATION

Figure 3-12. Hemothorax resulting from a closed chest injury.

3-24. TREAT A CASUALTY WITH TENSION PNEUMOTHORAX

A casualty with tension pneumothorax resulting from a closed chest injury should treated as soon as possible. A chest needle decompression should be performed. Maintain an open airway and assist with respiration if needed. Administer oxygen if available. Monitor the casualty for tracheal deviation or mediastinal shift.

3-25. CHECK FOR OTHER CONDITIONS

a. **Subcutaneous Emphysema.** Subcutaneous emphysema is caused by air from a damaged lung becoming trapped in the soft tissues of the chest wall. The trapped air forms little bubbles that cause a crackling sensation when palpated. A casualty with subcutaneous emphysema should be given respiratory support and evacuated.

b. **Pulmonary Contusion.** A pulmonary contusion is a bruise of the lung, usually caused by a blunt instrument or fall. Edema fluid and blood accumulates in the lung tissue. This accumulation interferes with the respiratory process and results in hypoxia (oxygen deficiency). A casualty with a pulmonary contusion should be given respiratory support and evacuated.

c. **Myocardial Contusion.** A myocardial contusion is a bruise of the heart muscle and is usually caused by a blunt injury to the chest. The casualty will have an irregular pulse with occasional pauses between heartbeats at times and a very rapid pulse at other times. A casualty with a suspected myocardial contusion should be evacuated immediately.

d. **Pericardial Tamponade.** Pericardial tamponade is caused by blood or other fluid accumulating in the pericardial sac that surrounds the heart. The fluid compresses the heart and interferes with its function. Pericardial tamponade is a life-threatening condition that requires respiratory support and immediate evacuation. Signs and symptoms of pericardial tamponade include the following.

    (1)   Very soft, faint heart sounds, which may be hard to hear even with a stethoscope.

    (2)   Congested and distended veins in the head and neck.

    (3)   Difficulty in breathing.

    (4)   Tachycardia (weak and rapid pulse).

    (5)   Rapidly decreasing blood pressure with the systolic and diastolic readings coming closer and closer together.

NOTE: The major differentiating factor between a tension pneumothorax and the pericardial tamponade is the presence or absence of breath sounds. In pericardial tamponade, the patient would still have equal and bi-lateral breath sounds.

e. **Massive Internal Bleeding.** Injury to the great blood vessels located within the chest can cause a rapid loss of blood. The casualty will show signs and symptoms of hypovolemic shock.

f. **Laceration of a Major Airway.** Injury to the trachea or bronchi can result in tension pneumothorax, hemoptysis (coughing up blood), and respiratory distress. Provide respirator support and evacuate the casualty. This patient will need immediate aggressive airway support that may not be feasible even during tactical field care.

g. **Abdominal Injuries.** Injuries to the lower ribs may indicate abdominal injuries, such as damage to the kidneys.

Continue with Exercises

EXERCISES, LESSON 3

INSTRUCTIONS: Answer the following exercises by marking the lettered response that best answers the question or best completes the sentence or by writing the answer in the space provided.

After you have answered all of the exercises, turn to "Solutions to Exercises" at the end of the lesson and check your answers. For each exercise answered incorrectly, reread the lesson material referenced with the solution.

1. Which of the following is a sign of an open chest wound?

    a. Blood being coughed up.

    b. Hissing sound coming from a chest wound.

    c. Bluish tint to the casualty's lips.

    d. All of the above are signs of an open chest wound.

2. The plastic envelope is placed directly over an open chest wound to:

    a. Prevent infection.

    b. Reduce blood loss.

    c. Keep air from going into the chest cavity.

    d. Keep the dressing from becoming contaminated.

3. If you find two open chest wounds (entry and exit wounds) when you examine the casualty, which wound should you seal and dress first?

    a. The larger wound.

    b. The smaller wound.

4. When treating a casualty with a sucking chest wound, have him

_____ and stop breathing when you put the plastic envelope

over the wound. Have him _____ and stop breathing when you
tie the tails of the field dressing in a knot.

5. What size of material should be used for making the airtight seal?

   a. Four inches by six inches.

   b. The sealing material should be larger than the wound and the distance
      between the edges of the sealing material and the edges of the wound
      should be two or more inches.

   c. The sealing material should be the same size as the wound.

   d. The sealing material should be slightly smaller than the size of the wound.

6. When applying the field dressing to an open chest wound, where should you tie
   the knot?

   a. Tie the knot at the edge of the dressing.

   b. Tie the knot directly over his spine.

   c. Tie the knot in the center of the dressing.

   d. Tie the knot on the uninjured side of the casualty's body.

7. You have treated a casualty with an open chest wound. His breathing had
   improved, but now his breathing is becoming difficult. He is short of breath and
   his lips are turning blue. What can you do to help the casualty?

   a. Nothing, the casualty's reactions are normal.

   b. Place a pressure dressing over the wound.

   c. Administer modified abdominal thrusts.

   d. Perform a chest needle decompression.

8. A casualty has a fractured rib. You should immobilize the fracture by:

   a. Taping the casualty's chest.

   b. Applying a sling and swathe to the arm on the casualty's injured side.

   c. Perform a and b above.

9. While palpating the chest area of a casualty with a suspected closed chest injury, you feel a crackling sensation almost as though you were pressing on tiny air bubbles. This is an indication of:

   a. Hemothroax.

   b. Myocardial contusion.

   c. Pericardial tamponade.

   d. Subcutaneous emphysema.

10. A puncture wound results in the casualty's left pleura cavity being penetrated. Which of the following statements is most likely to be true?

   a. The lungs will be unaffected.

   b. The right lung will rupture due to the sudden change in air pressure.

   c. The left lung will begin to collapse, but the right lung will still expand fully.

   d. Both lungs will collapse at the same time.

Check Your Answers on Next Page

SOLUTIONS TO EXERCISES, LESSON 3

1. d (paras 3-4a, f, j)

2. c (para 3-7b(5))

3. a (para 3-6)

4. Exhale, exhale. (paras 3-7a(6),b(3), d; 3-8b(3), (4)

5. b (para 3-7b(4)(b))

6. c (para 3-8b(4))

7. d (para 3-13)

8. b (para 3-16a; Caution)

9. d (para 3-25a)

10. c (para 3-3a)

End of Lesson 3

LESSON 4 Treating Abdominal Injuries.

TEXT ASSIGNMENT Paragraphs 4-1 through 4-14.

TLESSON OBJECTIVES When you have completed this lesson, you should be able to:

4-1. Identify the signs and symptoms of an abdominal injury.

4-2. Identify the procedures for treating a casualty with an open abdominal wound.

4-3. Identify the procedures for treating a casualty with an acute abdomen.

SUGGESTION Work the lesson exercises at the end of this lesson before beginning the next lesson. These exercises will help you accomplish the lesson objectives.

LESSON 4

TREATING ABDOMINAL INJURIES

Section I. GENERAL

4-1. ABDOMINAL CAVITY

The abdomen is a large body cavity that extends from the diaphragm to the pelvis. It contains several organs that are part of the digestive system, the urinary system, and the genital system. The liver, stomach, spleen, and intestines are some of the organs located in the abdominal cavity. Several large arteries and veins are also located in the cavity.

4-2. INJURIES TO THE ABDOMEN

Abdominal injuries may be closed (no skin broken) or open (skin broken and abdominal wall penetrated). Injuries to the genitalia may also be present. Injuries to the genitalia are not life-threatening, but are usually very painful. Treatment for these injuries will be conducted during the tactical field care phase of care.

a. **Open Abdominal Wounds.** Open abdominal wounds are caused by an object penetrating the skin and abdominal wall. The penetration may be caused by a bullet or a knife, by an object blown from an explosion, or by falling on a sharp object. Organs and/or blood vessels located in the abdominal cavity may be punctured. The wound may expose organs. Sometimes organs, such as part of an intestine, may protrude through the wound.

b. **Closed Abdominal Injuries.** Closed abdominal injuries are caused by a blow to the abdomen. Although the skin is not broken, organs and/or blood vessels located in the abdominal cavity may be lacerated or ruptured.

Section II. TREATING OPEN ABDOMINAL WOUNDS

4-3. LOCATE OPEN ABDOMINAL WOUND(S)

Examine the casualty's abdominal region for both entry and exit wounds. If more than one open abdominal wound is found, treat the most serious wound (largest or heaviest bleeding wound) first.

4-4. POSITION A CASUALTY WITH AN OPEN ABDOMINAL WOUND

After finding an open abdominal wound, position the casualty on his back with his knees raised in a flexed position (figure 4-1). This position helps to lessen pain, control shock, relieve pressure on the abdominal area by allowing the abdominal muscles to relax, and lessen exposure of abdominal organs.

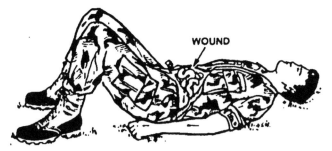

Figure 4-1. Casualty with an open abdominal wound positioned with his knees flexed.

4-5. TREAT FOR SHOCK

Treat the casualty for shock (Lesson 7). Even if the signs and symptoms of shock are not immediately present, performing measures to control shock should be your first concern. If heavy internal bleeding is not present and the organs are not perforated, the casualty's life is not in immediate danger from the injury itself. A casualty should be treated for shock whether he has an open or closed abdominal injury.

4-6. EXPOSE THE OPEN ABDOMINAL WOUND

Fully expose the wound area so you can see the full extent of the injury. Tear, cut, push, and/or lift the casualty's clothing from the area. Loosen any clothing or equipment that binds the casualty. Some special considerations are given in the following paragraphs.

a. **Chemical Environment.** If you are in a chemical environment, do not expose the wound as this would increase the casualty's exposure to the chemical agents. Dress the wound without further exposing the wound.

b. **Stuck Material.** If clothing or other material is stuck to the wound area, cut or tear around the stuck material. Do not remove the stuck material since removing the material might cause additional damage to the wound. Apply the envelope and dressing over the stuck material.

c. **Debris in Wound.** Do not try to clean the wound or remove objects or debris from the wound.

d. **Protruding Object.** If an object is protruding from the wound, do not remove the object. The impaled object is stabilized with bulky dressings after the dressing is applied to the wound.

e. **Protruding Organ (Evisceration).** Sometimes, part of an intestine or other organ is forced out through the wound. If an organ is outside the body, <u>do not</u> touch the exposed organ with your hands or try to push the organ back into the body. If the organ is lying outside the wound, use a dressing, T-shirt, or other clean, dry material to gently place the organ on top of the casualty's abdomen near the wound (not on the wound or in the wound). This is the accepted treatment for open abdominal wounds in combat.

NOTE: Other techniques include placing eviscerated organs back in to the abdominal cavity. These techniques are appropriate, but not thoroughly trained in this course. Once training on advanced techniques is obtained, these procedures may be utilized.

4-7.   APPLY A DRESSING

After you have exposed the wound and positioned any protruding organ, apply a dressing to the wound to help absorb the blood and protect the wound from additional contamination from the environment. If the injury is small, a field dressing is used. If the injury is large, an abdominal (ABD) dressing should be used. If an abdominal pad is not available, use an improvised dressing made from the cleanest materials available.

a. **Obtain a Dressing.** If the wound is small enough so only a field dressing is needed and the soldier still has a field dressing in his plastic individual first aid case, use his field dressing in order to conserve your supplies. If he does not have a field dressing available or if a larger dressing is needed, use a dressing from your aid bag.

b. **Open the Plastic Dressing Envelope.**

(1)   Use the bandage scissors from your aid bag to cut open the plastic envelope.

(2)   Remove the inner packet (abdominal dressing or field dressing wrapped in paper) and place the packet where it will not become contaminated.

(3)   Cut the other edges of the plastic envelope so the inside (sterile side) of the envelope can be applied to the wound. Avoid touching the inside surface of the plastic envelope and keep the inner surface as free from contamination as possible. Cut the envelope so as to not waste surface area needed to cover the wound.

c. **Apply the Plastic Envelope.** Place the envelope (sterile inner side down) over the wound and any protruding organ. The plastic will help to keep the eviscerated organ and other tissues from loosing moisture.

NOTE: Do not apply a plastic wrapper if it is contaminated or not large enough to cover the wound area.]

d. **Apply the Dressing to the Wound Area.** Open the paper-wrapped packet, remove the dressing from the paper wrapper, open the dressing, and place the white, sterile dressing pad over the plastic envelope.   Avoid touching the sterile part of the dressing.

(1)   If a plastic envelope was not applied to the wound, apply the dressing on top of the wound.

(2)   If an eviscerated organ is present, cover the wound and the organ. Apply a second dressing or improvised dressing, if needed.

(3)   If an object is protruding from the wound, dress the wound. Then improvise bulky dressings from the cleanest material available and build up the area around the object to stabilize the object. Do not cover the protruding object.

4-8.   SECURE THE DRESSING

Secure the dressing using the attached bandages. If improvised dressings are used, secure these dressings with cravats made from muslin bandages or with improvised bandages.

a. Hold the dressing in place with one hand to keep it from slipping while you are securing the dressing.

b. When taking a tail around the casualty, grasp the tail and slide it under the casualty. Reach down on the other side of the casualty, grasp the tail under the casualty, and pull.

c. Tie the tails in a non-slip knot at the casualty's side, not over the wound. The bandages should be tight enough to keep the dressing from slipping, but not tight enough to place excessive pressure on the injury. Pressure could cause additional damage to the organs of the abdominal cavity. The primary purpose of the dressing and bandages is to protect the wound from further contamination, not to control bleeding through pressure.

CAUTION: If an object is protruding from the wound, apply bandages to hold the bulky dressings in place. Do not wrap the bandages around the protruding object.

4-9.   DRESS OTHER OPEN ABDOMINAL WOUNDS, IF ANY

If there is more than one open abdominal wound, dress and bandage the other wound(s) in the same manner. If needed, improvise dressing and bandages from the cleanest material available.

4-10. REINFORCE DRESSING, IF NEEDED

Muslin bandages or improvised bandages made from strips torn from a T-shirt, blanket, or poncho may be applied over the dressings to add reinforcement. Make sure the reinforcing materials do not place undue pressure on the casualty's wound or on any protruding organs. Tie the reinforcing bandages at the casualty's side, but on the opposite side from the knot securing the dressing. Figure 4-2 shows reinforcing materials applied to an abdominal wound.

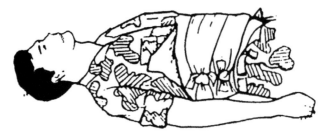

Figure 4-2. Reinforcing materials applied to an open abdominal wound.

4-11. MONITOR A CASUALTY WITH AN OPEN ABDOMINAL WOUND

a. Keep the casualty in the knees-up position.

b. Do not give the casualty anything to eat or drink. If the casualty complains of thirst, moisten his lips with a damp cloth.

c. Administer mouth-to-mouth resuscitation if the casualty stops breathing.

d. Record treatment on a U.S. Field Medical Card and attach the card to the casualty's clothing.

e. Evacuate the casualty.

f. Check the casualty's vital signs at least every 15 minutes if evacuation is delayed.

g. If you must leave the casualty, turn his head to one side. This will help promote drainage and help prevent choking should he vomit. Tell him to stay on his back and keep his knees up.

Section III. TREATING AN ACUTE ABDOMEN

4-12. CAUSES OF AN ACUTE ABDOMEN

The term "acute abdomen" is used to indicate the presence of any of a wide variety of abdominal disorders causing severe abdominal pain. An acute abdomen is usually accompanied by peritonitis, an inflammation of the peritoneum (the membrane lining the abdominal cavity). Peritonitis is usually caused by contents of a ruptured organ, such as the digestive juices and food from the stomach, fecal material from an intestine, urine from the bladder, bile from the liver, or pus from a ruptured appendix (appendicitis). It can also result from internal bleeding, disease, or contamination from an open abdominal wound. Peritonitis is always a danger with an open abdominal wound and often results from a closed abdominal injury.

4-13. SIGNS AND SYMPTOMS OF AN ACUTE ABDOMEN

    a. **Peritonitis.** Signs and symptoms of peritonitis include:

        (1)   Abdominal pain, local or diffused.

        (2)   Abdominal tenderness (palpate abdominal area).

        (3)   Tense (rigid), distended abdomen (palpate abdominal area).

        (4)   Rapid, shallow respirations.

        (5)   Tachycardia.

        (6)   Low blood pressure.

        (7)   Fever.

        (8)   Constipation.

        (9)   Nausea or vomiting.

        (10) Refusal of casualty to move, usually due to pain.

        (11) Referred pain (pain felt at a point other than the source of the pain).

b. **Internal Bleeding.** Internal bleeding into the digestive tract or abdominal region may be indicated by the following signs.

(1)   Blood being coughed up (hemoptysis).

(2)   Blood present in vomitus (hematemesis) or stools (hematochezia). (The blood may be bright red or dark due to interaction with digestive juices.)

(3)   Rigid abdominal cavity (cavity filled with blood).

4-14. TREATING A CASUALTY WITH AN ACUTE ABDOMEN

Place the casualty on his back with his knees flexed (paragraph 4-4). Treat the casualty for shock (Lesson 7). Maintain the casualty's airway and administer ventilations as needed. If the casualty vomits, perform a finger sweep to remove vomitus from his mouth. (If the vomitus is not removed, the casualty may inhale the vomitus and choke.) Administer oxygen (high percentage) if available. Do not allow the casualty to eat or drink anything. Do not administer any sedative or analgesic agent. If internal bleeding is present, keep the casualty as still as possible, initiate an intravenous infusion, and evacuate the casualty to a medical treatment facility immediately. Internal bleeding into a cavity cannot be controlled by the medic in the field.

Continue with Exercises

EXERCISES, LESSON 4

INSTRUCTIONS: Answer the following exercises by marking the lettered response that best answers the question or best completes the sentence or by writing the answer in the space provided.

After you have answered all of the exercises, turn to "Solutions to Exercises" at the end of the lesson and check your answers. For each exercise answered incorrectly, reread the lesson material referenced with the solution.

1. You are monitoring a casualty with an acute abdomen. How should the casualty be positioned?

   a. Flat on his back.

   b. On his back with his knees flexed.

   c. On his back with his feet elevated higher than the level of his heart.

   d. On his side with the uninjured side down.

2. If you find that the casualty has two abdominal wounds (entry and exit wounds), which wound should you treat first?

   a. The entry wound.

   b. The exit wound.

   c. The more serious wound.

3. A casualty has a small open abdominal wound. Which of the following is correct?

   a. You should begin treating the casualty for shock; then dress the open wound.

   b. You should dress the open wound; then treat for shock if signs and symptoms of shock develop.

   c. You should dress the open wound and ignore any signs and symptoms of shock.

4. A casualty has an open abdominal wound. A loop of intestine is protruding from the wound and lying on the ground. What should you do?

_____

_____

_____

_____

5. When securing the tails of a field dressing applied to an open abdominal wound, the bandages should be tied:

   a. Loose enough to avoid putting pressure on the wound but tight enough to keep the dressing in place.

   b. Tight enough to control the bleeding but not tight enough to stop blood circulation.

   c. As tightly as possible.

6. If you reinforce the abdominal dressings, where should you tie the knot of the reinforcing bandage?

   a. Directly over the wound.

   b. On the casualty's side, but not on the same side where the tails of the field dressing were tied.

   c. On the casualty's side next to the knot where the tails of the field dressing are tied.

7. Which of the following is/are correct procedures?

   a. If the plastic envelope from the field dressing is large enough to cover the wound and any eviscerated organs, apply the envelope (sterile side down) before applying the dressing.

   b. If an eviscerated organ is present, wash the organ with water from a canteen before you dress the wound.

   c. The procedures given in a and b are correct.

8. Which of the following should be treated for shock?

    a. A casualty with an open abdominal wound.

    b. A casualty with a closed abdominal injury with internal bleeding.

    c. A casualty with an acute abdomen.

    d. All of the above.

9. You have treated a casualty with an abdominal injury. The casualty says that he is hungry and thirsty. What should you do?

    a. Give the casualty something to eat and drink.

    b. Give the casualty something to drink, but nothing to eat.

    c. Give the casualty some fruit that will help to satisfy both his hunger and his thirst.

    d. Moisten the casualty's lips with a damp cloth, but do not give him anything to eat or drink.

Check Your Answers on Next Page

SOLUTIONS TO EXERCISES, LESSON 4

1. b (para 4-14)

2. c (para 4-3)

3. a (para 4-5)

4. Use clean material to pick up the intestine loop, place it on the casualty's abdomen, and cover the intestine and the wound with plastic and a dressing. (paras 4-6e; 4-7c, d)

5. a (para 4-8c)

6. b (para 4-10)

7. a (paras 4-6c, e; 4-7c, d)

8. d (paras 4-5, 4-14)

9. d (paras 4-11b, 4-14)

End of Lesson 4

LESSON ASSIGNMENT

LESSON 5   Treating Head Injuries.

TEXT ASSIGNMENT   Paragraphs 5-1 through 5-15.

LESSON OBJECTIVES When you have completed this lesson, you should be able to:

5-1.   Identify the signs and symptoms of open and closed head injuries.

5-2.   Identify the procedures for treating a casualty with an open head wound.

5-3.   Identify the procedures for treating a casualty with a closed head injury.

5-4.   Identify the procedures for treating a casualty with injury to the eye.

5-5.   Identify the procedures for treating a casualty with a nosebleed.

SUGGESTION   Work the lesson exercises at the end of this lesson before beginning the next lesson. These exercises will help you accomplish the lesson objectives.

LESSON 5

TREATING HEAD INJURIES

Section I. OPEN AND CLOSED HEAD INJURIES

5-1. GENERAL

A head injury may be the only injury (such as a single blow to the head from a blunt instrument) or it may be combined with other injuries (such as head and body injuries caused by an explosion). A head injury may consist of a cut of the scalp, a concussion, a contusion, a fracture of the skull with injury to the brain, or a combination of these injuries. If the skin has been broken, it is called an open head injury. If the skin has not been broken, it is a closed head injury. Both open and closed head injuries can be severe and life threatening.

5-2. IDENTIFY SIGNS OF AN OPEN HEAD WOUND

Bleeding from the scalp, visible skull fracture, and visible brain tissue are signs of an open head injury. You may not be able to evaluate the seriousness of a head injury by its appearance. A lacerated scalp may appear to be very serious due to profuse bleeding, but the bleeding can be controlled with a dressing. What appears to be a minor injury could be accompanied by injury to brain tissue that results in increased intracranial pressure, which can be fatal. The open wound may be a penetrating wound (entry wound with no exit wound) or a perforating wound (both an entry and an exit wound).

5-3. IDENTIFY SIGNS AND SYMPTOMS OF A CLOSED HEAD INJURY

Signs and symptoms of a closed head injury include the following.

a. Deformity of the head (skull fracture).

b. Clear or bloody fluid (cerebrospinal fluid) leaking from the nose and/or ear.

c. Periorbital discoloration ("black eyes" or "raccoon eyes").

d. Bruise behind one or both ears over the mastoid process (Battle's sign).

e. Slow pulse rate (may not be present if there is significant bleeding elsewhere).

f. Mental confusion or memory loss.

g. Staggering, dizziness, or drowsiness.

h. Increased intracranial pressure (paragraph 5-4).

5-4. IDENTIFY SIGNS AND SYMPTOMS OF INCREASED INTRACRANIAL PRESSURE

Increased intracranial pressure may be due to brain tissue swelling, blood or other fluid accumulating inside the skull, or to a combination of these situations. The following signs and symptoms may indicate increased intracranial pressure.

a. Headache.

b. Nausea and/or vomiting.

c. Loss of consciousness (either current or recent unconsciousness).

d. Dilated pupils that do not constrict when exposed to bright light (an early sign of serious head injury) or changes in pupil symmetry.

e. Lateral loss of motor nerve function in which one side of the body becomes paralyzed (may not occur immediately).

f. Slow respiratory rate or change in respiratory pattern.

g. A steady rise in the systolic blood pressure (may not be present if there is significant bleeding elsewhere).

h. A rise in the pulse pressure (systolic pressure minus diastolic pressure).

i. Elevated body temperature.

j. Restlessness (indicates insufficient oxygenation of the brain).

k. Slurred speech.

l. Convulsions or twitching.

m. Abnormal posturing.

Section II. TREATING OPEN HEAD WOUNDS

5-5. POSITION A CASUALTY WITH AN OPEN HEAD WOUND

After treating the casualty for any immediate life-threatening conditions, evaluate the casualty's condition and position him appropriately. The evaluation includes checking the casualty's level of consciousness using the AVPU method (alert, responds to verbal commands, responds to pain, unresponsive). The same rules are used to position a casualty after his open head wound has been dressed.

a. If the casualty has a suspected spinal fracture or severe head injury, do not move him unless it is necessary. Keep the casualty as immobile as possible while you dress his wound.

b. If the casualty is having convulsions (involuntary muscle movements such as uncontrolled jerking or shaking), gently support his head and neck to prevent the casualty from accidentally injuring himself. Do not try to forcefully hold his arms and legs. Trying to "pin down" jerking limbs will probably cause additional injury.

c. If the casualty is choking, nauseous, vomiting, or bleeding from his mouth, position the casualty on his side (figure 5-1) in the recovery position. This position is used since it promotes drainage and helps to maintain an open airway. Place the casualty on the side opposite that of the wound (wound away from the ground). Also place the casualty in this position if you must leave him.

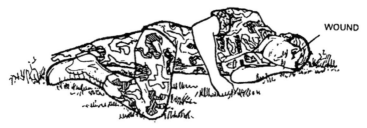

WOUND

Figure 5-1. Casualty with a minor open head wound positioned
on his side with the wound up.

5-6. TREAT AN OPEN HEAD WOUND

a. **Expose the Wound.** Remove the casualty's headgear to fully expose the wound.

CAUTION: If you are in a chemical environment and the "all clear" signal has not been given, do not remove the casualty's mask or hood and do not dress the wound. If the mask or hood has been breached, repair the breach with tape or wet cloth stuffing if possible.

b. **Replace Flap.** If the scalp is lacerated, there may be a skin flap. Replace the skin flap in its bed (area from which it was torn) before dressing the wound. Do not attempt to clean the wound or remove debris. Do not attempt to push any brain matter back into the head. If an object is protruding from the wound, do not remove the object. Stabilize the impaled object with bulky dressings when the wound is dressed.

c. **Dress the Wound.** Instructions for applying and securing field dressings to specific parts of the head are given in the following paragraphs. The dressing and bandages should not cover the casualty's eye or ear unless the eye or ear is injured. Reducing the casualty's vision or hearing could be dangerous in a combat situation.

NOTE: The procedures in paragraphs 5-7, 5-8, and 5-9 describe the use of a field dressing. The same techniques can be used with the emergency trauma dressing.

5-7.   APPLY A DRESSING TO A WOUND ON THE FOREHEAD OR BACK OF THE HEAD

The following paragraphs give instructions for applying a field dressing to a wound on the casualty's forehead. The same general procedures are used to dress a wound on the back of the casualty's head.

a. Remove the field dressing from its wrappers, grasp a tail in each hand, hold the dressing toward the wound, pull the dressing open, and place the sterile, white dressing pad on the wound.

b. Place one hand on the dressing to keep it from slipping. If the casualty is able, you can have him assist by holding the dressing in place.

c. Wrap one tail horizontally around the casualty's head (figure 5-2) and bring it back across the dressing. Angle the bandage so that it will cover the top or bottom edge of the dressing.

d. Wrap the second tail around the casualty's head in the opposite direction. Bring the tail back across the dressing angled so the tail will cover the other edge (top or bottom) of the dressing.

e. Continue to wrap the bandage around the head again until it meets the first tail.

f. Tie the tails in a non-slip knot on the side of the head (figure 5-3). The bandages should be tight enough so the dressing will not slip but not tight enough to place undue pressure on the wound.

g. Tuck in any excess tails. Tucking in excess material will keep the tails from catching on an object or accidentally hitting the casualty in the eye.

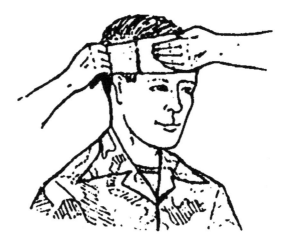

Figure 5-2. Wrapping a tail horizontally around the head
(wound on forehead).

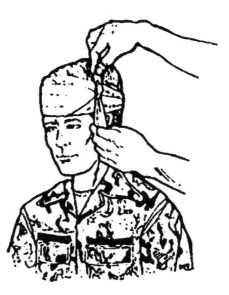

Figure 5-3. Tying the tails on the side of the head
(wound on forehead).

5-8. APPLY A DRESSING TO A WOUND ON THE TOP OF THE HEAD

a. Remove the field dressing from its wrappers, grasp a tail in each hand, hold the dressing directly over the wound, pull the dressing open, and place the white, sterile side of the dressing pad on the wound.

b. Place one hand on the dressing to keep it from slipping. If the casualty is able, you can have him assist by holding the dressing in place.

c. Grasp the near tail with the other hand.

d. Bring the tail down in front of the ear (figure 5-4), under the chin, up in front of the opposite ear, over the dressing, and to a point just above and in front of the first ear (about a one and one-fourth circle).

CAUTION: When passing a tail under the chin, make sure the tail remains wide and close to the front of the chin. This will keep the bandage from pressing against the casualty's trachea and interfering with his breathing.

e. Remove your hand from the dressing and grasp the other (free) tail.

f. Bring the second tail down the opposite side of the face in front of the ear, under the chin, and up until it meets the first tail (about a three-fourths circle).

g. Cross the tails so each makes a 90 degree turn. The cross should be made slightly above and in front of the ear.

h. Bring one tail across the casualty's forehead above the eyebrows until it is in front of the opposite ear (about a half circle). Bring the other tail back above the ear, low behind the head at the base of the skull, and up to a point above and in front of the opposite ear (about a half circle) where it meets the first tail (figure 5-5). Bringing the tail across the base of the skull keeps the bandage from slipping.

i. Tie the tails in a non-slip knot in front of and above the ear (figure 5-6) and tuck in any excess material.

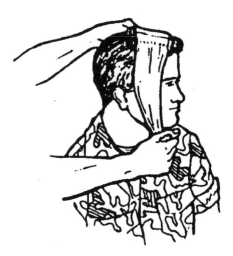

Figure 5-4. Bringing the tail under the chin
(wound on top of the head).

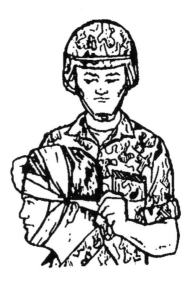

Figure 5-5. Crossing the tails
(wound on top of head).

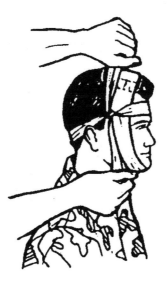

Figure 5-6. Tying the tails on the side of the head
(wound on top of head).

5-9. APPLY A DRESSING TO A WOUND ON THE CHEEK OR SIDE OF THE HEAD

a. Remove the field dressing from its wrappers, grasp a tail in each hand, hold the dressing in a vertical position with the white sterile side of the dressing toward the wound, pull the dressing open, and place the dressing pad on the wound (figure 5-7).

b. Place one hand on the dressing to keep it from slipping. If the casualty is able, you can have him assist by holding the dressing in place.

c. Bring the top (uppermost) tail over the top of the head, down in front of the ear on the uninjured side, under the chin, up the side of the face, and over the dressing to a point just above the ear (a full circle). Make sure the tail remains wide and close to the front of the chin when passing under the chin.

d. Bring the other tail down, under the chin, up the uninjured side in front of the ear, and over the top of the head until it meets the first tail.

e. Cross the two tails just above the ear on the injured side of the head (figure 5-8).

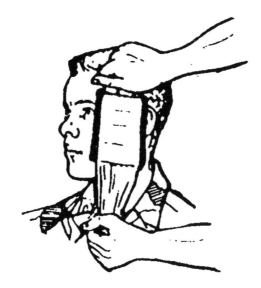

Figure 5-7. Placing the dressing pad over the wound
(wound on cheek).

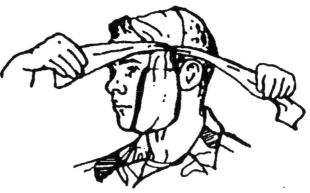

Figure 5-8. Crossing the tails
(wound on cheek).

f. Bring one tail across the forehead (above the eyebrows) to a point just in front of the opposite ear (the ear on the uninjured side of the head). Bring the other tail above the ear, low behind the back of the head at the base of the skull, and above the other ear until it meets the first tail.

g. Tie the tails in a non-slip knot just above and in front of the ear on the uninjured side of the head (figure 5-9). Tuck in the ends of the tails.

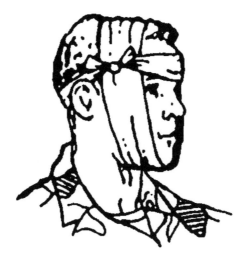

Figure 5-9. Tails tied in a non-slip knot and ends tucked (wound on cheek).

5-10. MONITOR A CASUALTY WITH AN OPEN HEAD WOUND

Position the casualty (paragraph 5-5). Continue to check the casualty's level of consciousness every 15 minutes. If the casualty falls asleep, wake the casualty to check his level of consciousness. Be aware of any changes in the casualty's condition. Reposition the casualty, if needed. Maintain the casualty's airway, if needed. Do not give the casualty anything to eat or drink since eating or drinking could cause the casualty to vomit. Treat the casualty for shock, if needed. If the wound is serious (other than a minor scalp laceration), provide oxygen (if available) and evacuate the casualty.

Section III. TREATING OTHER INJURIES

5-11. TREAT A CASUALTY WITH A SEVERE HEAD INJURY

About one in ten casualties with a head wound who are unconscious also have a spinal injury. If a casualty has a fractured spine, the sharp edge of a fractured bone could damage or sever the spinal cord. Always assume the casualty has a spinal fracture if he is unconscious or has signs of a severe head wound such as a fractured skull or clear or bloody cerebrospinal fluid leaking from the nose or ear. If a spinal injury is suspected, do not move the casualty unless you must move him to save his life. For example, you would move the casualty (and yourself) out of a burning building or position the casualty for mouth-to-mouth resuscitation if he is not breathing and lying on his abdomen.

a. Immobilize any casualty with a suspected spinal injury. Subcourse MD0533, Treating Fractures in the Field, gives procedures for immobilizing a casualty with a suspected spinal fracture.

b. If an open head wound is present, dress the wound to protect it from further contamination. Do not apply pressure to the wound.

c. If cerebrospinal fluid is leaking from an ear, apply a loose field dressing to the ear using the procedures for applying a dressing to the side of the head (paragraph 5-9). Cover the ear with the dressing. The dressing will absorb the drainage and help to protect the area from additional injury and contamination. If there is also drainage from the other ear, pass the tails over the ear so they will provide protection to that ear also.

5-12. TREAT A CASUALTY WITH A CLOSED HEAD INJURY

A closed head injury may be serious even if there does not appear to be a fracture of the skull or spinal injury. A casualty with a closed head injury should be evaluated by a medical officer. Monitor a casualty with a closed head injury. Continue to check the casualty's level of consciousness every 15 minutes and take vital signs. Evacuate the casualty if signs and symptoms of increased intracranial pressure are noted.

5-13. TREAT A CASUALTY WITH AN INJURY TO THE EYE

Brief descriptions of treatments for some eye injuries are given in the following paragraphs. If the casualty is wearing contact lenses, do not attempt to remove them. Evacuate a casualty with any of the described injuries. Additional information is given in Subcourse MD0547, Eye, Ear, and Nose Injuries.

a. **Impaled Object.** If an object is embedded in the eye, place dressings around the object to keep it stable. Cover both eyes with bandages. Covering the uninjured eye helps to keep the uninjured eyeball still. If the uninjured eyeball moves, the injured eyeball will also move. If the injured eyeball moves, additional injury may occur.

b. **Lacerations.** If an eye has lacerations, place a light, sterile dressing over the eye. Then place a shield or cup over the injured eye and cover both eyes with bandages. Avoid putting pressure on the eye.

c. **Extruded Eyeball.** If an eyeball is extruded (popped out of its socket), do not attempt to replace the extruded eyeball. Place bulky dressings around the eye, cover the extruded eyeball with a moist dressing, and place a paper cup or cone over the eye to protect the eyeball. Bandage both eyes.

5-14. TREAT AN UNCONSCIOUS CASUALTY

a. Monitor the casualty's breathing. Keep the airway open and perform rescue breathing or cardiopulmonary resuscitation, if needed. Cardiopulmonary resuscitation is not indicated in the tactical situation when other casualties would benefit from treatment efforts. Insert a Combi-tube airway to protect the casualty's airway.

b. Initiate an intravenous infusion, if needed.

c. Continue to check the casualty's level of consciousness (AVPU or Glascow Coma Scale [GCS] method) and vital signs every 15 minutes. Observe for signs and symptoms of increased intracranial pressure.

d. Evacuate the casualty.

e. If you must leave the casualty, position him so he will not aspirate vomitus should vomiting occur. If the casualty is lying in a prone position, make sure his head is turned to one side. Otherwise, position the casualty on his side as shown in figure 5-1. Keep the casualty's head, neck, and back in alignment when repositioning the casualty. Place padding such as a rolled poncho or a folded field jacket around the casualty to support the casualty and maintain spinal alignment.

5-15. TREAT A CASUALTY WITH A NOSEBLEED

A nosebleed (epistaxis) may cause a loss of blood sufficient to result in shock. The blood seen flowing from the nose may not be a true indication of the amount of bleeding that is occurring since most of the blood may flow into the throat and be swallowed. Sometimes the blood can block the casualty's airway or be aspirated.

a. **Causes of Epistaxis.** A nosebleed can be caused by a blow to the face or head (possible skull fracture), infection such as sinusitis, high blood pressure, digital trauma to the nasal airway, and certain diseases.

b. **Treating Epistaxis.** A nosebleed can be controlled using the following procedures.

(1) Position the casualty in a sitting position with his head tilted forward. This position helps the blood to drain through the nose rather than entering the throat.

(2) Apply pressure to the nostrils. Pressure can be applied by pinching the nostrils together. Pressure can also be applied by placing a rolled piece of gauze bandage between the upper lip and gum; then pressing the bandage against the nasal region with the fingers.

(3) Apply an ice pack or ice wrapped in material to the nose. The local cooling will help to control the bleeding.

(4) Keep the casualty calm and quiet. Anxiety may cause an increase in blood pressure that may cause an increase in bleeding.

c. **Monitoring the Casualty.** If bleeding cannot be stopped or if the bleeding reoccurs, a more serious injury (such as posterior pharyngeal bleeding) may be present. Evacuate the casualty to a medical treatment facility. Treat the casualty for hypovolemic shock if needed and provide oxygen if available.

Continue with Exercises

EXERCISES, LESSON 5

INSTRUCTIONS: Answer the following exercises by marking the lettered response that best answers the question or best completes the sentence or by writing the answer in the space provided.

After you have answered all of the exercises, turn to "Solutions to Exercises" at the end of the lesson and check your answers. For each exercise answered incorrectly, reread the lesson material referenced with the solution.

1. You are treating a casualty who was injured in an explosion. The casualty is unconscious and unresponsive. He has a bruise behind one ear and a slightly bloody fluid is leaking from that ear. There is a depressed area on that side of the casualty's head, but the skin is not broken and the injury is not bleeding. His pulse rate and respiratory rate are slow. You should suspect the casualty has:

   a. A possible spinal injury.

   b. A closed head injury.

   c. An open head wound.

   d. A closed head injury with possible spinal injury.

2. A casualty has an open head wound on his forehead just above his left eye. He is conscious and does not appear to have any other significant injury. After you dress his wound, he states that he feels like he may throw up. How should you position the casualty?

   a. Have the casualty lie on his chest.

   b. Have the casualty lie on his right side.

   c. Have the casualty lie on his left side.

   d. Have the casualty lie on his back with his feet elevated.

3. When treating a casualty with an open head wound in a chemical environment, you should:

   a. Remove the casualty's protective gear, dress the wound, and replace the protective gear.

   b. Repair any damage to the protective gear and not dress the wound until the "all clear" has been given.

4. You are applying a field dressing to a casualty with an open head wound on the top of his head. Where should you tie the tails in a non-slip knot?

   a. On top of the casualty's head, directly over the wound.

   b. On the side of the casualty's head.

   c. Under the casualty's chin.

5. You have to leave a casualty who has an open wound on the right side of his head. The casualty is drowsy and cannot sit up. How should you position the casualty?

   a. On his back with his feet elevated.

   b. On his back with his head raised.

   c. On his left side.

   d. On his right side.

6. A soldier has suffered a blow to the head. He is conscious and does not have any fractures or open wounds. He does, however, have some bloody fluid draining from his left ear. What should you do?

   a. Cover the left ear with a field dressing.

   b. Apply a pressure dressing to the left ear.

   c. Position the casualty on his left side to promote the drainage. No dressing is needed.

7. When monitoring a casualty with a head injury, you should reevaluate

   the casualty's level of consciousness every _____.

8. Which of the following statements is/are true?

   a. A minor nosebleed can often be controlled by rolling up a gauze pad, placing the pad under the casualty's upper lip, and pressing the pad against the nasal region with the fingers.

   b. A nosebleed that does not respond to pressure or which reoccurs may indicate a more serious injury.

   c. A nosebleed can result in a blocked airway.

   d. All of the above statements are correct.

Check Your Answers on Next Page

SOLUTIONS TO EXERCISES, LESSON 5

1. d (paras 5-3, 5-4, 5-12)

2. a (para 5-6d)

3. b (para 5-7 Caution)

4. b (para 5-9i)

5. c (paras 5-6c, 5-15e)

6. a (para 5-12c)

7. Fifteen minutes. (paras 5-11, 5-13, 5-15c)

8. d (paras 5-15, 5-15b(2), c)

End of Lesson 5

LESSON 6	Treating Burns.
TEXT ASSIGNMENT	Paragraphs 6-1 through 6-28.
LESSON OBJECTIVES	When you have completed this lesson, you should be able to:

6-1.   Identify signs and symptoms of thermal, electrical, chemical, and radiant energy burns.

6-2.   Identify the procedures for smothering flames.

6-3.   Identify the procedures for treating a casualty with a thermal burn.

6-4.   Identify the procedures for removing a casualty from an electrical wire.

6-5.   Identify the procedures for treating a casualty with an electrical burn.

6-6.   Identify the procedures for treating a casualty with a chemical burn.

6-7.   Identify the procedures for treating a casualty with a radiant energy burn.

6-8.   Identify the procedures for treating a casualty with a burn to the eye.

SUGGESTION   Work the lesson exercises at the end of this lesson before beginning the next lesson. These exercises will help you accomplish the lesson objectives.

LESSON 6

TREATING BURNS

Section I. GENERAL

6-1. TREATING A CASUALTY WITH BURNS

When you first discover the burn casualty, stop the burning process if the casualty is still being burned in order to protect both the casualty and yourself. Once this has been done, continue to perform your evaluation of the casualty. Exactly when the burn wound is treated depends on the seriousness of the burn injury and on other injuries that the casualty may have suffered. A burned area on a fractured limb should be dressed and bandaged before a splint is applied to the limb. Minor burns on a casualty with a life-threatening injury may not be treated until the casualty reaches a medical treatment facility.

6-2. TYPES OF BURNS

Burns can be classified by their cause. Burns can result from thermal (heat), electrical, chemical, or radiant (laser) sources. Burns can also be classified by the degree (depth) of the burn.

6-3. DETERMINING THE DEGREE OF BURN

Burns can be classified by the depth of the burn (the number of damaged tissue layers). A burn can be a first-degree burn, a second-degree burn, or a third degree burn. Different areas may be burned to a different degree. A third degree burn may be surrounded by an area of second-degree burns that, in turn, may be surrounded by first-degree burns.

a. **Skin Layers.** The skin consists of three primary layers, the epidermis, the dermis, and the subcutaneous tissue (figure 6-1). Beneath the subcutaneous layer is the fascia. The fascia covers the muscles that lie beneath the skin.

(1) Epidermis. The epidermis is the outer layer of the skin. This layer consists of dead cells that are constantly being rubbed off and replaced from beneath. The epidermis contains no blood vessels or nerves, but does contain the pigments that give the skin color.

(2) Dermis. The dermis (true skin) layer lies under the epidermis. The dermis contains sweat glands, sebaceous (oil) glands, hair follicles, small blood vessels (but not major blood vessels), and specialized nerve endings.

(3) <u>Subcutaneous tissue</u>. The subcutaneous tissue lies beneath the dermis and is composed primarily of fat. The fat serves as an insulator against cold temperatures.

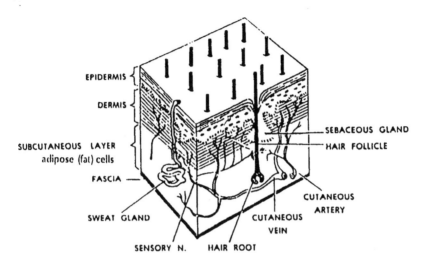

EPIDERMIS

DERMIS

SEBACEOUS GLAND

SUBCUTANEOUS LAYER
adipose (fat) cells

HAIR FOLLICLE

FASCIA

CUTANEOUS ARTERY

SWEAT GLAND

CUTANEOUS VEIN

SENSORY N.   HAIR ROOT

Figure 6-1. Skin layers.

b. **Degrees (Depth) of Burn.**

(1) <u>First-degree burns</u>. First-degree burns cause the skin to be red and painful (like a sunburn), but does not produce blisters. It involves only the superficial skin (epidermis).

(2) <u>Second-degree burns</u>. Second-degree burns are more serious. The burn is painful and blisters are present. There is damage to the epidermis and the dermis. There may also be some swelling in the subcutaneous layer even though the layer is not actually damaged.

(3) <u>Third-degree burns</u>. Third-degree burns involve damage to or destruction of all three layers of skin. It usually involves damage to the fascia and may also include damage to underlying muscles, nerves, blood vessels, and/or bone. The skin may look leathery, dry, and discolored (charred, brown, or white). Clotted blood vessels may be visible under the burned area and subcutaneous fat may be visible. Third degree burns may not be painful because the nerves have been destroyed, but the surrounding area with second and first-degree burns may be painful. Third-degree burns involve a large loss of body fluid that can lead to shock.

Section II. TREATING THERMAL BURNS

6-4. IDENTIFY THE SOURCE OF A THERMAL BURN

Thermal burns are caused by heat. They can be caused by contact with a flame, a hot object, hot liquid, hot gas (such as steam), or the fireball from a nuclear explosion.

6-5. REMOVE SOURCE OF THE BURN, IF PRESENT

Remove the source of the burn if it is still present (put out flames, wash off hot liquid with cool water, remove casualty from steam, and so forth). If the casualty's clothing is on fire, have the casualty stop, drop to the ground, and roll on the flames until they are out. Do not allow a casualty to run as this will only fan the flames. If the casualty remains standing, the flames may ignite his hair and/or be inhaled.

a. If possible, cover the casualty with a large piece of nonsynthetic material, such as a wool or cotton blanket, and roll the casualty on the ground until the flames are smothered (figure 6-2). Do not use synthetic materials because synthetic material may melt and cause additional injury.

b. If a source of water is readily available, douse the flames with water.

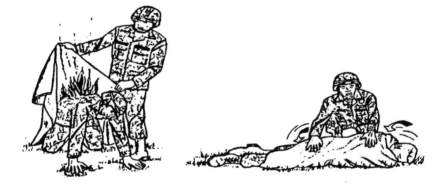

Figure 6-2. Smothering flames.

6-6. CHECK FOR INHALATION INJURY

Inhaling heated air can damage the respiratory system. Check for respiratory distress and maintain an open airway, if needed. Continue to monitor the casualty's respirations closely since 30 to 40 minutes may elapse before edema obstructs the airway and causes respiratory distress. Signs of inhalation injury include the following.

  a. Facial burns.

  b. Singed eyebrows, singed eyelashes, and/or singed nasal hairs.

  c. Carbon deposits and/or redness in the mouth or throat.

  d. Sputum containing sooty carbon.

  e. Hoarseness, noisy inhalation, or brassy sounding cough.

  f. Difficulty in breathing (dyspnea).

6-7. CHECK FOR CARBON MONOXIDE POISONING

If the casualty was inside a burning building or other closed structure, he may have carbon monoxide poisoning. Signs and symptoms of carbon monoxide poisoning include the following.

NOTE: Carbon monoxide (CO) is formed when materials burn without sufficient oxygen being present. When carbon monoxide is inhaled, some red blood cells bond with the carbon monoxide instead of oxygen (O_2). This results in a decrease of oxygen in the blood system since the body cannot use carbon dioxide like it does oxygen. A casualty suffering from carbon should be given oxygen if it is available.

  a. Dizziness and/or headache.

  b. Nausea.

  c. Cherry-red colored skin and mucous membranes (check the lining inside the casualty's lips). This is a late sign.

  d. Rapid pulse (tachycardia).

  e. Rapid breathing (tachypnea).

  f. Respiratory distress, including possible respiratory arrest.

NOTE: Pulse oximeters are not effective on carbon monoxide poisoning patients. They will falsely read 100 percent due to the carbon monoxide binding to the hemoglobin.

6-8. EXPOSE THE BURNED AREA

Remove all smoldering clothing and objects that retain heat. Cut and gently lift away any clothing covering the burned area. Do not pull clothing over the burned area.

CAUTION: Do not cool the burned area with water on any burn greater than 10 percent body surface area. Over cooling of any burn can cause the patient to become rapidly hypothermic.

CAUTION: Do not immerse a third degree burn.

a. **Stuck Clothing.** If clothing is stuck to the burned area, cut around the clothing and do not disturb the stuck clothing.

b. **Jewelry.** If the casualty is wearing jewelry on a burned arm or hand, remove the jewelry and put it in his pocket. Burns often cause swelling and the jewelry may have to be cut off later if it is not removed now. Tell the casualty what you are doing and why.

c. **Chemical Environment.** If you are in a chemical environment, do not expose the wound. Apply the dressing over the protective garments.

6-9. ESTIMATE THE PERCENT OF BODY SURFACE AREA BURNED

An estimate of the percent of body surface burned is used to determine if fluid replacement (intravenous infusion) is needed to prevent or help control shock and, if so, the amount of fluid to be administered. The amount of body surface burned can be estimated using the "rule of nines." The approximate skin surface of each section of an adult body is shown in figure 6-3.

a. When estimating the amount of skin surface burned to determine the amount of intravenous fluids to be administered, only count the areas covered by second-degree and/or third-degree burns.

b. If the casualty is a small child, the percentages change slightly. Figure 6-4 gives the approximate body surface area (BSA) percentages for a small child.

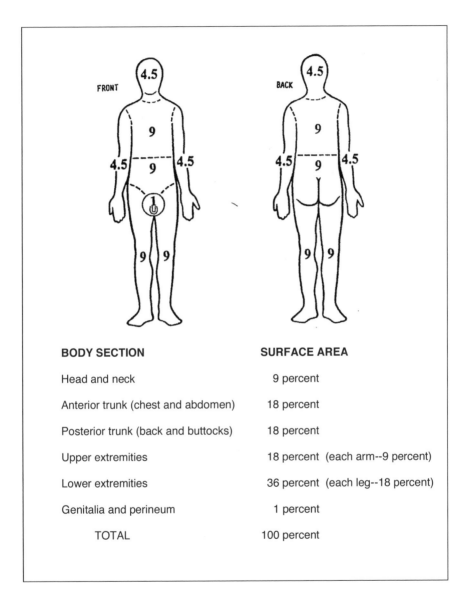

BODY SECTION

SURFACE AREA

Head and neck   9 percent

Anterior trunk (chest and abdomen)   18 percent

Posterior trunk (back and buttocks)   18 percent

Upper extremities   18 percent (each arm--9 percent)

Lower extremities   36 percent (each leg--18 percent)

Genitalia and perineum   1 percent

TOTAL   100 percent

Figure 6-3. Rule of nines for an adult casualty.

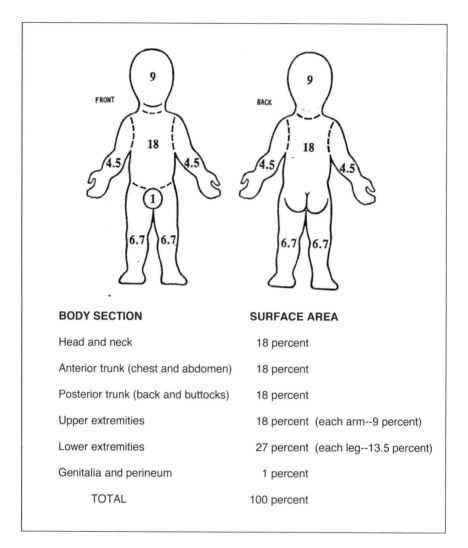

BODY SECTION	SURFACE AREA
Head and neck	18 percent
Anterior trunk (chest and abdomen)	18 percent
Posterior trunk (back and buttocks)	18 percent
Upper extremities	18 percent (each arm--9 percent)
Lower extremities	27 percent (each leg--13.5 percent)
Genitalia and perineum	1 percent
TOTAL	100 percent

Figure 6-4. Rule of nines for a small child.

6-10. INITIATE AN INTRAVENOUS INFUSION, IF NEEDED

Burns result in a loss of body fluid even if there is no observed bleeding. If 20 percent or more of the casualty's body is covered with second- and third-degree burns, initiate an intravenous infusion (IV) to help prevent or control hypovolemic shock. Early signs of hypovolemia in a burn patient indicate internal hemorrhaging or other hemorrhaging. Re-evaluate the casualty for indications of hemorrhage.

a. Keep the casualty flat on his back.

b. Determine the amount of fluid to infuse and the flow rates.

(1) Estimate the casualty's weight in kilograms (kg). (A casualty's weight in kilograms can be determined by dividing his weight in pounds by 2.2. Figure 6-5 can be used to convert the casualty's approximate weight in pounds to kilograms.

Pounds	Kilograms	Pounds	Kilograms	Pounds	Kilograms
88	40	187	85	286	130
99	45	198	90	297	135
110	50	209	95	308	140
121	55	220	100	319	145
132	60	231	105	330	150
143	65	242	110	341	155
154	70	253	115	352	160
165	75	264	120	363	165
176	80	275	125	374	170

Figure 6-5. Table for converting pounds to kilograms.

(2) Multiply the casualty's weight (in kilograms) by the percent of body surface area burned (paragraph 6-9).

(3) Multiply the product obtained in step (2) by 4. The resulting figure is the amount of replacement fluid in milliliters (same as cubic centimeters) that should be administered to the casualty over a 24-hour period.

(4) Divide the amount by two. The result is the number of milliliters (ml) which the casualty should receive during the first 8 hours. The remaining amount is administered during the remaining 16 hours.

(5) Divide the quotient obtained in step (4) by 8 to determine the amount of IV fluid to be administered per hour during the first eight hours. Divide the quotient obtained in step (4) by 16 to determine the amount of IV fluid to be administered per hour during the remaining 16-hour period.

(6) Divide the amount per hour by 60 to determine the amount per minute.

(7) Multiply the amount per minute by the number of drops per milliliter (usually 10 drops equal one milliliter) to obtain the number of drops per minute to be administered. This is the flow rate. Note that the flow rate (drops per minute) for the first eight hours is twice as fast as the flow rate (drops per minute) for the last 16 hours.

(8) An example is given in figure 6-6.

c. Select a large peripheral vein for needle insertion.

(1) If possible, initiate the IV in an area which has not been burned. An accessible vein with overlying burned skin can still be used, however.

(2) A vein in an upper extremity is usually preferred over a vein in a lower extremity.

d. Select a large gauge (16 gauge or 18 gauge) needle.

e. Initiate the intravenous infusion using the procedures given in Subcourse MD0552, Injections and Intravenous Infusions. Ringer's injection lactated (RL) is the preferred replacement fluid. Normal saline (NS) is the second fluid of choice.

An adult casualty weights 165 pounds. He has second- and third-degree burns over his back, buttocks, and the backs of both legs. Compute the flow rate for the first 8 hours; then for the remaining 16 hours if 10 drops equal one milliliter.

1. Estimate BSA burned:
Back--	9 percent
Buttocks --	9 percent
Back of left leg --	9 percent
Back of right leg --	9 percent
Total --	36 percent

2. Estimate weight in kilograms
   165 pounds/2.2 pounds per kilogram = 75 kilograms

3. Multiply weight (kg) by the percent of body surface area burned
   75 x 36 = 2700   (Note: The percent BSA is not a decimal.)

4. Multiply by 4 milliliters.
   2700 x 4 ml = 10,800 ml (total fluid for first 24-hour period)

5. Divide by 2.
   10,800 ml/2 = 5400 ml   (total fluid administered during first 8 hours; total fluid administered during following 16 hours)

6. Divide first half by 8.   Divide second half by 16.
   5400 ml/8 hours = 675 ml per hour (first 8 hours)
   5400 ml/16 hours = 337.5 ml per hour (remaining 16 hours)

7. Divide by 60.
   675/60 = 11.25 ml per minute (first 8 hours)
   337.5/60 = 5.625 ml per minute (remaining 16 hours)

8. Multiply by the number of drops per milliliter
   11.25 x 10 = 112.5 drops per minute (first 8 hours)
   5.625 x 10 = 56.25 drops per minute (remaining 16 hours)

   NOTE: Drops per minute figure will be rounded when actually setting IV flow rate.

Figure 6-6. Example of a flow rate computation using modified Brook formula for calculating replacement fluid.

6-11. APPLY COLD SOAKS, IF APPROPRIATE

If the casualty has second-degree burns on 10 percent or less of his body surface (no third degree burns) and the situation allows, cool the area with running water. Do not soak or immerse the effected area in water since this will promote bacteria growth.

a. Do not cool for more than 10 minutes. Prolonged cooling can result in hypothermia.

b. Do not apply cooling to third-degree burns. This could increase the risk of infection.

c. Do not apply cooling to extensive burns (over 10 percent BSA burned).

d. Do not place the casualty's body in a tub of water. Hypothermia could result.

6-12. DRESS THE BURN WOUNDS

Apply dry, sterile dressings over the burned areas. If the burned area is too large to cover with regular dressings, cover the burned area with a sterile sheet, clean linen, or the cleanest material available.

a. Do not try to clean the burned area before applying the dressings.

b. Do not place dressings over burns of the face or genitalia.

(1) If the eye area is burned, the burned eyelids will swell to protect the underlying eye. Protect the eyes from exposure to light.

(2) If the eye area is burned, the casualty is to be evacuated immediately, If materials are readily available, a loose, sterile gauze dressing moistened with sterile saline may be placed over each eye.

c. Do not break any blisters that have formed.

d. Do not apply any grease or ointment to the burned areas.

6-13. MONITOR AND EVACUATE THE CASUALTY

Continue to perform your evaluation and treat other injuries. Evacuate the casualty, if needed. Some considerations are given below.

a. **Administer Oxygen, if Needed and Available.** If the casualty has signs and symptoms of inhalation injury or carbon monoxide poisoning, administer humidified oxygen at a high flow rate if it is available. Be very aggressive in monitoring the casualty for deterioration of the airway. Be prepared to administer artificial ventilations and manage the airway, if needed.

b. **Adjust IV Flow, if Needed.** If an intravenous infusion has been started and you are able to measure urine output, adjust the IV fluid flow to maintain an average urine output between 30 and 60 milliliters per hour. Urine output is a reliable guide to assess circulating blood volume. As long as renal artery pressure remains above 90 mm Hg (millimeters of mercury), urinary output should remain adequate.

c. **Monitor Pulse Sites in Extremities.** Check the casualty's circulation by checking the distal pulse site in each arm and leg.

d. **Allow Casualty to Drink, if Appropriate.** If the casualty is not in shock and is not nauseated, you can give him small sips of cool water to drink. Stop administering the water if the casualty feels as though he may vomit or if signs or symptoms of shock develop.

e. **Evacuate the Casualty.** A casualty with inhalation injury or carbon monoxide poisoning needs to be evacuated as soon as possible. Burns of the throat can swell and impair breathing. Swelling in a burned extremity can have a tourniquet-like effect on blood circulation in the extremity.

Section III. TREATING ELECTRICAL BURNS

6-14. IDENTIFY THE SOURCE OF AN ELECTRICAL BURN

Electrical burns are caused by an electrical current passing through the body. They can be caused by coming into contact with a charged ("live") electrical wire, lightning, or other source of electrical energy.

6-15. SEPARATE THE CASUALTY FROM THE ELECTRICAL SOURCE

If the casualty is still in contact with the source of the electrical current, such as lying on a "live" electrical wire, separate the casualty from the source of the current. Assume that any electrical wire is alive (carrying electrical current) and is a danger to you as well as to the casualty.

a. **Stop the Current, if Practical.** If the electrical current can be turned off quickly, such as flipping a nearby switch, turn off the current first. If it will take more time to turn off the current than to separate the casualty from the electrical wire, cut off the electrical current after you have removed the casualty from the current and have treated the casualty.

CAUTION: Assume the electrical wire is still carrying electrical current even though you think you turned off the current. Do not touch the electrical wire or the casualty as long as he is in contact with the wire. Electrical current can pass from the wire through the casualty to you.

b. **Separate Casualty and Current.** You must separate the casualty from the current before beginning your evaluation of the casualty. Either remove the wire from the casualty or remove the casualty from the wire. If rubber gloves are readily available, put them on before moving the wire or casualty.

(1)   Move the wire away from the casualty. Stand on a dry surface. Loop a dry rope, dry clothing, or other material which will not readily conduct electricity under the casualty's body and lift the casualty from the wire. Have a second person use a wooden limb or similar nonconductor to move the wire away from the casualty (figure 6-7). Gently lower the casualty to the ground after the wire has been removed.

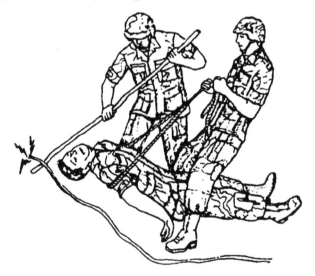

Figure 6-7. Removing an electrical wire beneath a casualty.

(2) Move the casualty away from the wire. If you cannot remove the wire from the casualty (no other soldier available to assist, for example), remove the casualty from the wire. Loop material that will not readily conduct electricity, such as a dry rope, around the casualty's limb and drag the casualty away from the wire. Do not let your body come into contact with the casualty or the wire during the process.

6-16. CHECK FOR BREATHING

Electrical shock often renders the casualty unconscious and causes difficulties in breathing and heartbeat. If the casualty is unresponsive, open his airway and check for breathing. If the casualty is not breathing, check his pulse.

a. If no pulse is present, perform cardiopulmonary resuscitation.

b. If a pulse is present, administer mouth-to-mouth resuscitation. Continue to check for a pulse every 12 breaths.

c. If the casualty resumes breathing on his own, continue with your evaluation.

CAUTION: Never attempt to administer mouth-to-mouth resuscitation until the wire and the casualty have been separated.

6-17. LOCATE ENTRY AND EXIT BURNED AREAS

Electrical burns can be deceiving. The burn may not appear to be serious because only a small area of skin is burned. In reality, however, a great deal of damage may have been done to the interior of the casualty's body. Electrical burns involve both an entry burn where the current entered the body and an exit burn where the current left the body. An exit burn may appear on any part of the body and can be in a quite different location from the entry burn. The sole of the foot is a common location for the exit burn.

6-18. EXPOSE THE BURNED AREAS

Cut and gently lift away any clothing covering the burned area.

a. Do not pull clothing over the burned area.

b. Cut around any stuck clothing and apply the dressing over the burned area and stuck clothing.

c. If the casualty is wearing jewelry on a burned arm or hand, remove the jewelry in case the limb swells. Put the jewelry in the casualty's pocket.

6-19. DRESS THE BURNED AREAS

Apply dry sterile dressings over the entry and exit burned areas. The dressings will help to prevent contamination and control any bleeding from the wounds. Tie the tails tight enough to hold the dressing in place, but not tight enough to put undue pressure on the injury. Follow the general rules given in paragraph 6-12.

6-20. TREAT SHOCK AND EVACUATE THE CASUALTY

If signs and symptoms of hypovolemic shock are present, initiate an intravenous infusion. Take other measures to control shock. Evacuate the casualty to a medical treatment facility.

Section IV. TREATING CHEMICAL BURNS

6-21. IDENTIFY THE SOURCE OF THE CHEMICAL BURN

Chemical burns are caused by contact with either liquid or dry chemicals. Most burns are caused by a reaction between the chemical and the casualty's body. Examples of such chemicals include ammonia, caustic soda, quick-lime and white phosphorus (WP). White phosphorus is a chemical used in marking rounds and grenades that begins to give off heat and light when exposed to air.

NOTE: Burns caused by blister agents are covered in Subcourse MD0534, Chemical, Biological, Radiation, Nuclear, Explosives.

6-22. REMOVE CHEMICALS FROM THE SKIN

Chemicals that attack the skin will continue to burn the skin as long as the chemical is in contact with the skin. Chemicals should be removed as soon as possible.

a. **Liquid Chemicals.** If the burn is caused by a liquid chemical, pour as much water as possible over the burned area. (This is called "flushing" the area.) Use cool water from a canteen, Lyster bag, or water trailer if it is available. If a sufficient amount of water is not available, use any nonflammable fluid to flush the area.

(1) Flush the area for at least 20 minutes. Flush longer if the chemical is an alkali, such as caustic soda. Alkalies penetrate deeper and cause more severe injuries.

(2) Do not delay flushing in order to remove the casualty's clothing. Remove his clothing and jewelry while flushing the area.

(3) Do not use a hard blast of water to flush the burned area. High water pressure can increase the damage to the tissues.

(4) Some chemicals have a delayed reaction. Flush even though the casualty does not feel pain. Do not stop flushing just because the casualty's pain goes away.

b. **Dry Chemicals.** If the chemical is in a dry form (such as lime), use a clean, dry cloth to brush off loose particles of the dry chemical. Take care to avoid getting the particles on your body. After brushing off the particles, flush the area with as much water or other nonflammable liquid as possible.

CAUTION: If a large amount of water or other nonflammable liquid is not available, do not flush the area until the casualty has been moved to an area where sufficient water is available. Applying a small amount of water to a dry chemical may cause a chemical reaction which transforms the dry chemical into an active, burning substance. Do not attempt to irrigate the area unless you can continue flushing for at least 20 minutes.

c. **White Phosphorus.** White phosphorus becomes active (burns) when exposed to air. It sticks to the skin and continues to burn until it is deprived of air. White phosphorus usually causes multiple, deep second- and third-degree burns.

(1) Quickly smother the flame with a non-petroleum liquid such as water, mud, or urine. If possible, submerge the entire area in water.

(2) If possible, remove the particles of white phosphorus from the skin. This can be accomplished by brushing the skin with a wet cloth and/or using forceps, a knife, or similar instrument to remove the particles.

(3) If the particles cannot be removed, cover the area with wet cloth or mud. The wet material or mud will keep air from getting to the white phosphorus and, thus, keep the particles from beginning to burn again.

CAUTION: Do not use grease or oil on a white phosphorus burn. Grease or oil may cause the body to absorb the poisonous white phosphorus particles.

d. **Radioactive Fallout.** Burns caused by radioactive particles sticking to the casualty's skin are treated by brushing the particles from the casualty and flushing the skin with water. Take care to keep the radioactive particles and contaminated water from coming into contact with your skin and clothing.

6-23. REMOVE CHEMICALS FROM AN EYE

Chemicals such as acid, alkali, and petroleum can destroy the tissues of the eye. Chemicals can cause pain, redness, watering or tearing, and erosion of the surface of the cornea of the eye. Some chemicals may stick to the eye. If chemicals are in the casualty's eye, the eye must be flushed with potable (drinkable) water as quickly as possible. If possible, use sterile water or sterile saline (sterile saline is preferable since it will cause less pain to the patient) to flush the eye. Fluid from an IV bag (with tubing connected), water from the casualty's canteen, or water from a shower can be used. Do not try to neutralize the chemical in the eye.

a. **Chemicals in Only One Eye.**

(1) Turn the casualty's head to one side with the eye to be flushed (irrigated) lower than the other eye. This keeps chemicals from the eye being flushed from flowing into the other (unaffected) eye.

(2) Gently hold the casualty's eyelids open.

(3) Gently pour the water into the eye. Pour from the inner canthus (where the eyelids come together; closest to the nose) to the outer canthus (where the eyelids come together; closest to the side of the head).

(4) Continue to flush the eye with water for at least 5 minutes. If the chemical is an alkali (such as lye), flush for at least 20 minutes.

b. **Chemicals in Both Eyes.**

(1) Have the casualty lie down with his face up.

(2) Turn the casualty's head slightly to one side.

(3) Gently hold the eyelids of the casualty's lower eye open and begin flushing the eye. Pour from the inner canthus to the outer canthus. Turning the head and pouring from the inner to outer canthus help to keep contaminated water from entering the other eye.

(4) Turn the casualty's head slightly to the other side.

(5) Gently hold the eyelids of the casualty's lower eye (eye not just flushed) open and begin flushing that eye, pouring from the inner edge of the eye to the outer edge.

(6) Continue to alternate flushing one eye, then the other. Continue to flush both eyes for at least 5 minutes (20 minutes if the chemical is an alkali).

6-24. DRESS THE BURNED AREAS

a. **Skin.** After the chemicals have been removed from the casualty's skin, apply dry, sterile dressings over the burned areas with the exceptions listed below. Do not break any blisters or apply any ointment.

(1) Do not place dressings over burns of the face or genitalia.

(2) If white phosphorus particles are still present, cover the burn with a moist cloth, mud, or other substance that will keep the white phosphorus from having contact with the air.

b. **Eye(s).** If chemicals have been flushed from an eye, cover the eye with a clean, sterile dressing.

6-25. TREAT FOR SHOCK, IF NEEDED, AND EVACUATE THE CASUALTY

If signs and symptoms of hypovolemic shock are present, initiate an intravenous infusion and take necessary measures to control shock. Evacuate the casualty to a medical treatment facility.

Section V. TREATING RADIANT ENERGY BURNS

6-26. IDENTIFY THE SOURCE OF THE RADIANT ENERGY BURN

Radiant energy injuries are caused by bright, visible light (such as lasers and electric welding arcs) or by forms of light energy that are not visible (such as ultraviolet and infrared light). Sunburn is a type of radiant energy burn caused by exposure to the sun's ultraviolet rays. Microwave radiation caused by electromagnetic radiation is also a type of radiant energy. The primary danger of radiant energy is damage to the eyes.

a. **Laser Beam.** A laser (light amplification by stimulated emission of radiation) beam may be visible or invisible, depending upon the frequency of the beam. Laser devices include range finders, target designators, and weapon guidance systems (SMART missiles and bombs). Lasers are also used in communications centers and in weapons simulation training, such as MILES (multiple integrated laser engagement system). The primary danger is to the eye since the eye focuses and concentrates whatever light enters the eye. Lasers can cause temporary or permanent damage to one or both eyes. Minor interference with vision can reduce the casualty's ability to aim his weapon, drive his vehicle, or read a map. Some laser devices may be powerful enough to produce burns on exposed skin. Signs and symptoms of laser injury include the following.

(1)   Reduced vision in one or both eyes.

(2)   Seeing a bright flash of light just before the reduced vision.

(3)   Pain. (Some injuries cause eye discomfort, but most injuries produce no pain.)

(4)   A feeling of heat within the eyes.

(5)   Burns to the cornea and/or hemorrhaging within the eyeball.

(6)   Skin burns ranging from redness to surface charring to deep tissue damage around the eye.

NOTE: For additional information on laser injury, read Field Manual 8-50, Prevention and Medical Management of Laser Injuries.

b. **Welding Arc.** A person who looks directly at a welding arc can receive burns on the surface of his eyes that can result in severe pain and sensitivity to light. The pain and sensitivity to light may last two or three days until the burn has healed. Mild symptoms may appear even if the person did not look directly at the welding arc. Signs and symptoms include the following.

(1)   Gritty feeling in the eyes.

(2)   Severe pain.

(3)   Immediate decrease in vision.

(4)   Inability to tolerate light.

(5)   Redness.

(6)   Swelling around the eye.

(7)   Watering or tearing.

c. **Microwave Radiation.** Microwaves are used by radar and communication systems. The primary danger is damage to the eyes, especially damage that results in cataracts. Microwaves can also interfere with production of red blood cells and can result in temporary sterility in males. Signs and symptoms of exposure to microwave radiation include the following.

(1)   Nausea.

(2)   Difficulty in swallowing.

(3) Hearing problems.

(4) Irritability or euphoria due to effects on the central nervous system.

(5) Whole body heating (hyperthermia).

6-27. TREAT A CASUALTY WITH A RADIANT ENERGY BURN

a. **Prevent Additional Damage to Eyes.**

(1) Protect the soldier from additional exposure to the radiant energy source. Keep the casualty from looking at the light source or remove him from the path of the radiation. If the radiant energy burn was caused by a light source, have the casualty don protective goggles. Special protective goggles are available to protect the wearer's eyes from specific wavelengths of light commonly used by laser devices.

(a) Other soldiers should also don protective goggles if they have not already done so.

(b) Sunglasses provide some protection if goggles are not available.

(2) Keep the casualty out of bright sunlight.

(3) Tell the casualty to not squeeze his eyelids. The pressure could cause additional damage.

b. **Apply Ointment, If Appropriate.** If the cornea has been damaged (burned) by a laser and the eye has not been perforated, apply antibiotic ointment to the injured eye.

c. **Cover the Eye, If Appropriate.**

(1) If the cornea has been burned by a laser, apply a patch to the injured eye. If only one eye is injured, do not apply a patch to the uninjured eye.

(2) Do not cover the casualty's eye if the cornea is not burned and he must see to perform his combat duties. If the casualty does not need to use his vision (does not need to walk or continue his mission), he may feel more comfortable if a cloth or loose bandage is placed over both eyes.

d. **Perform Other Measures as Needed.**

(1) Administer analgesic pain relief as needed.

(2) Treat any burns on exposed skin around the eye as thermal burns.

(3)   Reassure the casualty that you will take care of him. Reduced vision, even if no pain is present, may present serious psychological problems. Most casualties will have little or no permanent damage to their sight.

6-28. MONITOR AND EVACUATE THE CASUALTY

a. If you are in a combat situation, return a casualty who had a temporary loss of vision with no pain and no visible damage to the eye to duty. Evacuate a casualty with pain, visible damage to the eye, or vision problems that do not improve to a medical treatment facility.   Evacuate the casualty in a supine position.

b. If you are not in a combat situation, evacuate the casualty to a medical treatment facility for further evaluation by a medical officer.

NOTE: The evacuation is usually by ground ambulance since the injury does not justify aeromedical evacuation.

Continue with Exercises

EXERCISES, LESSON 6

INSTRUCTIONS: Answer the following exercises by marking the lettered response that best answers the question or best completes the sentence or by writing the answer in the space provided.

After you have answered all of the exercises, turn to "Solutions to Exercises" at the end of the lesson and check your answers. For each exercise answered incorrectly, reread the lesson material referenced with the solution.

1. A dry chemical has blown into a soldier's left eye and he is in pain from the burning sensation. What should you do?

    a. Turn his head so his left eye is lower than the right eye and flush the left eye with water.

    b. Turn his head so his left eye is higher than the right eye and flush the left eye with water.

    c. Turn his head so his left eye is lower than the right eye and flush both eyes with water.

    d. Turn his head so his left eye is higher than the right eye and flush both eyes with water.

2. A soldier has second-degree and third-degree burns covering one complete leg (front and back of lower leg and thigh) and his abdomen (lower half of the anterior trunk). Approximately how much of his body surface area has second- and third-degree burns?

    a. 18 percent.

    b. 27 percent.

    c. 36 percent.

    d   54 percent.

3. You should initiate an IV on a casualty if ___ percent or more of his body surface area (BSA) is covered with _____ and/or _____ degree burns.

4. You have examined a thermal burn casualty and estimate that 36 percent of his body surface area is covered with second and third degree burns. The casualty weighs about 175 pounds. You cannot evacuate the casualty due to the military situation. Using the formula given in this subcourse, what volume of intravenous fluid should the casualty receive per hour during the first eight hours?

   a. Around 6300 milliliters per hour.

   b. Around 2880 milliliters per hour.

   c. Around 1580 milliliters per hour.

   d. Around 720 milliliters per hour.

   e. Around 360 milliliters per hour.

5. Assuming 10 drops per milliliter, the flow rate for exercise 4 would be about ____ drops per minute.

6. A burn in which the skin is red but no blisters are present is a:

   a. First-degree burn.

   b. Second-degree burn.

   c. Third-degree burn.

7. You are in a chemical environment and find a soldier with a thermal burn to the side of his chest. You should:

   a. Expose the burned area, apply ointment or grease to the burned area, and apply a field dressing.

   b. Expose the burned area and apply a field dressing.

   c. Apply a field dressing to the burned area without further exposing the wound.

   d. Leave the burned area exposed to the air.

8. You and another soldier are going to remove an electrical wire from a soldier lying on top of the wire. Which of the following should you use to move the wire?

    a. A metal pole.

    b. A wooden pole.

9. Look for entry and exit wounds if the casualty has a(n) _____ burn.

10. Which of the following burns can properly be covered with mud?

    a. Electrical burn.

    b. Radiant energy burn.

    c. Thermal burn.

    d. White phosphorus burn.

11. Which of the following is a proper treatment for a soldier who was exposed to a laser beam, but who has suffered no damage to the cornea?

    a. Apply antibiotic ointment to the injured eye.

    b. Cover the casualty's eyes with bandages even if he needs his vision to perform critical combat duties.

    c. Keep the casualty out of bright sunlight.

    d. Tell the soldier to close his eyes and squeeze his eyelids as tight as possible.

12. A soldier has suffered third-degree burns over most of his arm. Should you immerse the arm in water from a lake to help reduce the excess heat in the arm?

    a. Yes, but not for more than 15 minutes.

    b. No, the danger of infection is too great.

13. The back of a soldier's shirt has caught on fire. You have no non-synthetic material to cover the soldier. You should:

    a. Roll him on the ground until the flames go out.

    b. Have him lie on his stomach until the flames go out.

    c. Have him stand up and pat the flames out with your hands.

    d. Cover him with synthetic material and roll him on the ground.

Check Your Answers on Next Page

SOLUTIONS TO EXERCISES, LESSON 6

1. a   (para 6-23a)

2. b   (figure 6-3; leg = 18 percent, abdomen = 9 percent (half of posterior trunk); 18+9=27)

3. 20 (twenty); second, third. (para 6-10)

4. d   (paras 6-10b(1) through b(5); figures 6-5, 6-6)

   175 lbs / 2.2 lb per kg = 80 kg (rounded)
   80 x 36 = 2880
   2880 x 4 = 11,520 ml (volume for first 24-hour period)
   11,520 ml / 2 =5760 ml (volume for first 8-hour period)
   5760 ml / 8 hr= 720 ml/hr (volume per hour for first 8-hour period)

5. 120. (paras 6-10b(6), b(7); figure. 6-6)

   720 ml per hour / 60 minutes per hour = 12 ml per minute
   12 ml/min x 10 drops/ml = 120 drops per minute

6. a   (para 6-3b(1))

7. c   (para 6-8c)

8. b   (para 6-15b(1))

9. Electrical. (para 6-17)

10. d   (paras 6-22c(3), 6-24a(2))

11. c   (para 6-27a(2))

12. b   (para 6-11b)

13. a   (para 6-5)

End of Lesson 6

LESSON ASSIGNMENT

LESSON 7   Treating Hypovolemic Shock.

TEXT ASSIGNMENT   Paragraphs 7-1 through 7-8.

LESSON OBJECTIVES   When you have completed this lesson, you should be
                          able to:

                          7-1.   Identify the signs and symptoms of hypovolemic
                                  shock.

                          7-2.   Identify procedures for preventing and treating
                                  hypovolemic shock.

                          7-3.   Given a situation, determine whether or not
                                  medical anti-shock trousers should be used.

                          7-4.   Identify the procedures for applying and inflating
                                  medical anti-shock trousers.

SUGGESTION   Work the lesson exercises at the end of this lesson
                          before beginning the next lesson. These exercises will
                          help you accomplish the lesson objectives.

LESSON 7

TREATING HYPOVOLEMIC SHOCK

7-1. IDENTIFY THE CAUSES OF SHOCK

Shock exists when the circulatory system fails to provide sufficient circulation to parts of the body. Organs and tissues that do not receive sufficient fluids (blood and plasma) fail to perform due to inadequate cellular perfusion. There are several types of shock. Any significant injury causes some degree of shock. It may be slight and unnoticed, lasting only a moment, or it may be severe enough to cause death.

a. **Hypovolemic Shock.** Hypovolemic shock results when there is a decrease in the volume of circulating fluids in the body. Hypovolemic shock is usually caused by severe bleeding (hemorrhaging) or severe loss of body fluids (dehydration) due to heat injury, severe burns (second- and third-degree burns on 20 percent or more of the body surface area), vomiting, diarrhea, or excessive sweating.

b. **Other Types of Shock.** The following are types of shock that also result in inadequate cellular profusion.

(1) Metabolic shock. Metabolic shock is caused by a severe fluid loss due to an illness.

(2) Neurogenic shock. Neurogenic shock is caused by dilation of the blood vessels due to loss of nervous control over the vascular system. There is not enough blood and plasma in the circulatory system to fill the vessels even though no circulatory fluids have been lost.

(3) Psychogenic shock. Psychogenic shock (fainting) is caused by a temporary dilation of the blood vessels which results in a decreased blood supply to the brain.

(4) Cardiogenic shock. Cardiogenic shock is caused by a failure of the heart to pump sufficient blood.

(5) Septic shock. Septic shock is caused by a severe infection that attacks the blood vessels and causes them to loose circulating fluid.

(6) Respiratory shock. Respiratory shock is due to an insufficient amount of oxygen in the blood.

(7) Anaphylactic shock. Anaphylactic shock is caused by an allergic reaction to an insect sting, food, drugs, or other substance. In anaphylactic shock, the casualty's skin may be flush, warm, itch, or break out. The face and tongue may swell and the lips turn bluish (cyanosis). The casualty may have difficulty in breathing, cough, or have pain in the chest. The blood pressure drops and pulse becomes weak, which results in faintness or coma.

7-2. IDENTIFY SIGNS AND SYMPTOMS OF HYPOVOLEMIC SHOCK

Severe loss of blood is the primary cause of hypovolemic shock. Other indications (signs and symptoms) of hypovolemic shock include:

a. Restlessness and anxiety.

b. Weak and rapid (thready) pulse.

c. Cool, clammy (sweaty) skin.

d. Profuse sweating (diaphoresis).

e. Pale skin color and/or blotchy or bluish skin around the mouth.

NOTE: In casualties with dark skin, check the color of the mucous membranes on the inside of the mouth.

f. Shallow, labored, rapid, or irregular breathing or gasping for breath.

g. Dull eyes with dilated pupils.

h. Excessive thirst.

i. Nausea or vomiting.

j. Gradual and steady drop in blood pressure.

k. Mental confusion.

l. Loss of consciousness.

7-3. TAKE MEASURES TO PREVENT OR TREAT HYPOVOLEMIC SHOCK

When the casualty has received an injury that may result in shock (such as severe external or internal bleeding or severe burns), take measures to prevent shock from developing. Do not wait until the signs and symptoms of shock appear before beginning to take action. The measures used to help prevent shock from occurring are also used to treat shock once it has developed. Perform the following measures when you suspect shock will develop or has already occurred.

a. **Reassure Casualty.** Reassure the casualty that you will take care of him. This should help to calm the casualty and reduce his anxiety. Anxiety increases the heart rate, which makes the casualty's condition worse.

b. **Maintain Airway.** Make sure that the casualty's airway remains open. Use the head-tilt/chin-lift or jaw thrust, if needed. Administer oxygen if it is available.

c. **Control Bleeding.** Take measures to control external and internal bleeding.

d. **Initiate IV.** Initiate an intravenous infusion with Ringer's lactate or normal saline to replace lost fluid. Select a large gauge (16 gauge or 18 gauge) needle.

(1) When fluid loss is due to bleeding, use small fluid bolus to return the casualty's peripheral pulses and mental status.

(2) When fluid loss is due to burns, compute the flow rate as shown in Lesson 6.

e. **Position the Casualty to Help Control Shock.** If the casualty has not already been placed in normal shock position (figure 7-1), place him in that position unless his condition dictates otherwise. If the casualty is on a litter, elevate the foot of the litter.

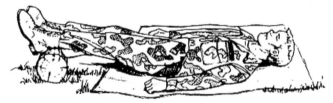

Figure 7-1. Casualty in the normal shock position.

CAUTION: If the casualty has a suspected spinal injury, immobilize his head, neck, and back using the procedures given in Subcourse MD0533, Treating Fractures in the Field. Do not elevate his legs.

CAUTION: If the casualty has an abdominal injury, leave the casualty on his back with his knees flexed (Lesson 4).

(1)   Position the casualty on his back. If possible, place a poncho or blanket under the casualty to protect him from the ground.

(2)   Check for fractures of the lower extremities and splint any fractures found. Do not elevate the legs until all lower limb fractures have been splinted.

(3)   Elevate the casualty's legs so his feet are slightly higher than the level of his heart. This helps the blood in the veins of his legs to return to his heart.

(4)   Place a small log, field pack, box, rolled field jacket, or other stable object under the casualty's feet or ankles to maintain the elevation.

(5)   If the casualty is unconscious, turn his head to one side so fluids can drain from his mouth.

f. **Loosen the Casualty's Clothing.** Loosen any binding clothing, including boots. Tight clothing can interfere with blood circulation. Avoid rough handling during the process.

CAUTION: Do not loosen or remove the casualty's protective clothing in a chemical environment.

g. **Maintain Casualty's Body Temperature.**

(1)   In warm weather, keep the casualty in the shade. If natural shade is not available, erect an improvised shade using a poncho and sticks or other available materials. It is better to keep the patient slightly warm rather than cool. A patient that is cool is losing body heat and is therefore at risk for hypothermia.

(2)   In cool weather, cover the casualty with a blanket, poncho, or other available materials to keep him warm and dry (figure 7-2). Place covering under the casualty to prevent chilling due to contact with cold or wet ground.

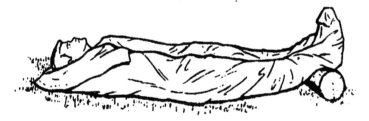

Figure 7-2. Protecting a shock casualty from cool temperatures.

7-4. MONITOR A CASUALTY FOR HYPOVOLEMIC SHOCK

Continue to monitor the casualty as you continue your evaluation and treatment. If the casualty is able, he may drink water. Do not give any thing by mouth to a patient who is nauseous, vomiting, or has an altered mental status.

a. **Monitor Vital Signs.** Continue to take the casualty's vital signs every 5 minutes until they return to normal; then take his vital signs every 15 minutes. Check the casualty's capillary refill by pressing on his nails and observing the return of color to the nail beds.

b. **Monitor Level of Consciousness.** Check the casualty's level of consciousness every 5 to 15 minutes as you monitor his vital signs.

c. **Monitor IV Flow Rate.** If the casualty's blood pressure stabilizes with the return of peripheral pulses, discontinue the IV and monitor the patient.

d. **Record Treatment.** Initiate a U.S. Field Medical Card on the casualty. Record treatment procedures and vital signs on the card.

e. **Apply Pneumatic Counterpressure Device (PCPD), If Applicable.** If the casualty is not responding to treatment for shock, medical anti-shock trousers (MAST) are available, and their use is appropriate (paragraph 7-5), apply them using the procedures given in paragraphs 7-6 through 7-8. Medical anti-shock trousers are usually found in a battalion aid station or other medical treatment facility.

NOTE: There is more than one type of MAST device. The MAST devices are also called military anti-shock trousers.

7-5. DETERMINE IF MEDICAL ANTI-SHOCK TROUSERS SHOULD BE USED

Medical anti-shock trousers can be applied to a casualty showing signs and symptoms of hypovolemic shock when the casualty is not responding to treatment for shock or when the cause of shock is not known. The MAST can also be used to help control internal bleeding in the abdomen or legs and to stabilize a fracture of the pelvis. Some general rules for deciding if the MAST should be applied are given below.

a. The MAST can be used if the casualty has one of the following conditions and no contraindications exist.

(1) Systolic blood pressure reading is less than 60 mmHg and other signs and symptoms of hypovolemic shock are present. (The systolic is the higher number of a blood pressure reading.)

(2)   Closed abdominal injury with signs and symptoms of hypovolemic shock present with systolic is less than 90 mmHg.

(3)   Pelvic fracture(s) with signs and symptoms of hypovolemic shock present and with systolic less than 90 mmHg.

b. Do not apply the MAST if one of the following conditions (contraindications) exist.

(1)   The casualty has psychogenic, anaphylactic, cardiogenic, or septic shock. (The MAST is used only with hypovolemic shock.)

(2)   The casualty has an injury that will be aggravated by applying the MAST. (For example, you should not apply the MAST to a casualty with an impaled object protruding from a wound in the leg or intestine protruding from an open abdominal wound unless you are ordered to do so by a physician.)

(3)   The casualty has congestive heart failure.

c. Do not apply the MAST to a casualty with one of the following conditions unless you are directed to do so by a physician.

(1)   The casualty has a severe head injury.

(2)   The casualty has an open chest wound or bleeding into the chest cavity.

(3)   The casualty has other trauma above the level of the MAST application.

(4)   The casualty is in heart failure with pulmonary edema.

(5)   The casualty may have an aortic aneurysm.

7-6.   PLACE THE MEDICAL ANTI-SHOCK TROUSERS ON THE CASUALTY

If use of the MAST is appropriate, apply the device and prepare to inflate the MAST.

NOTE: There are several different MAST models. Follow the manufacturer's instructions for applying, inflating, deflating and maintaining the MAST. You should be able to open the kit, position the MAST, and inflate the legs (paragraphs 7-6 and 7-7) within 90 seconds.

a. **Open the Kit.** Open the MAST kit and remove the MAST (inflatable leg and abdominal sections) and the accessories (pump and hoses).

b. **Unfold the Medical Anti-Shock Trousers .** Unfold the MAST and unfasten the Velcro clos Unfold the MAST so the left leg overlaps the right leg. Make sure the outside Velcro fasteners face the ground and the valves are on the outside next to the ground.

c. **Position the Medical Anti-Shock Trousers.**

(1) If there is sufficient space below the casualty's feet, lay the MAST out flat with the leg sections in the same direction as the casualty's legs (trousers in same relative position as casualty's pants).

(2) If there is not sufficient space below the casualty's feet, lay the MAST flat beside the casualty with the leg sections in the same direction as the casualty's legs. Position the top of the MAST abdominal section just below the casualty's lowest rib. If the casualty is very short, roll up the ends of the leg sections at the ankles.

(3) If the terrain is rough and a backboard is available, lay the MAST flat on the backboard. The backboard can remain in place when you position the MAST under the casualty.

d. **Prepare the Casualty.** Check for sharp objects in the casualty's pants and gear. Remove these objects before applying the MAST. Remove or cut away restrictive or bulky clothing or gear that could prevent the MAST from stabilizing the casualty.

e. **Place the Medical Anti-Shock Trousers Under the Casualty.** Have another soldier assist you put the MAST beneath the casualty. Serious injury or discomfort can result if the casualty has a pelvic injury or a traction splint and one person tries to apply the MAST alone. The steps given below can be used for a MAST placed below the casualty's feet or beside the casualty. If your assistant is not a medical person, you should lift the casualty while the assistant slides the MAST in position. Figure 7-3 shows two medics applying the MAST.

CAUTION: Do not lift the casualty any higher than absolutely necessary. If a spinal injury is suspected, use the log roll technique described in Subcourse MD0001, Evacuation in the Field, and Subcourse MD0533, Treating Fractures in the Field.

(1) Lift the casualty's legs high enough to slide the MAST underneath.

(2) Slide the MAST under the casualty's legs and up to the buttocks area.

(3) Lift the casualty's buttocks high enough to slide the MAST underneath.

(4)   Slide the top portion of the MAST under the casualty's buttocks and waist (figure 7-3). Position the top of the abdominal section just below the casualty's lowest rib.

f.   **Wrap the Casualty's Leg.** Either of the casualty's legs may be wrapped first, but the left leg is usually wrapped first.

(1)   Bring the left top part of the MAST across the casualty's abdomen and bring the outer part of the left trouser leg over the casualty's left leg (figure 7-4).

(2)   Smooth the MAST leg around the casualty's left leg.

(3)   Align the Velcro strips.

(4)   Bring the inside part of the left trouser leg over the outer part of the trouser leg (the part lying on top of the casualty's leg).

(5)   Press the Velcro strips of the left trouser leg firmly together to secure the seam of the trouser leg (figure 7-5).

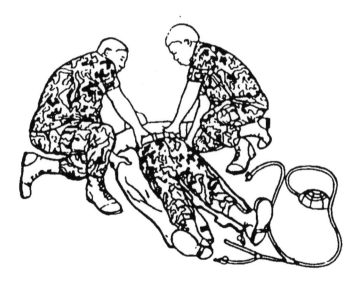

Figure 7-3. Positioning the MAST underneath the casualty.

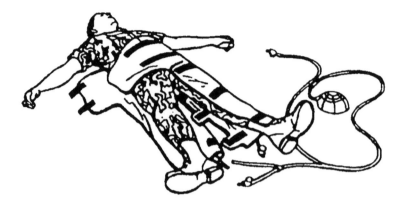

Figure 7-4. Wrapping the MAST around the casualty's leg.

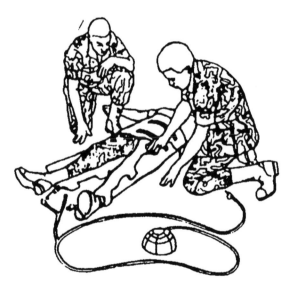

Figure 7-5. Securing one leg of the MAST.

g. **Wrap the Casualty's Other Leg.** Wrap the right trouser leg around the casualty's right leg using the same procedures given in paragraph f.

h. **Wrap the Casualty's Abdomen.**

(1) Bring the right top part of the MAST across the casualty's abdomen and over the part already lying on the casualty's abdomen.

(2) Align the Velcro strips.

(3) Press the Velcro strips firmly together to secure the abdominal portion of the MAST (figure 7-6).

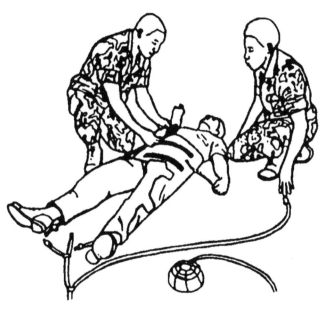

Figure 7-6. Securing the abdominal section of the MAST.

7-7. INFLATE THE MEDICAL ANTI-SHOCK TROUSERS

Once the MAST has been positioned around the casualty's legs and abdomen, it must be inflated to apply the desired pressure.

a. **Connect Hoses.** The foot pump has an air hose attached. The tube ends in a "Y" connector which has two other tubes attached, one short and the other longer. The shorter tube ends in another "Y" connector with two tubes attached. The tubes connected to the second "Y" are used to inflate the legs of the MAST. The longer tube from the first "Y" is used to inflate the abdominal section of the MAST. The foot pump and the hoses are shown in figures 7-4, 7-5, and 7-6.

(1)   Connect the end of one of the short tubes to the tube attached to one of the legs of the MAST (figure 7-7). Use a twisting motion when connecting the tubes.

(2)   Connect the end of the other short tube to the tube attached to the other leg of the MAST. Use a twisting motion when connecting the tubes. The air tubes will now look like figure 7-8.

(3)   Connect the remaining long tube to the tube attached to the abdominal section of the MAST. Use a twisting motion when connecting the tubes.

b. **Open Stopcock Valves.** There are three stopcock (inflation/deflation) valve knobs on the MAST that control airflow. One stopcock valve knob is located on the tube attached to the right trouser leg and another is located on the tube attached to the left trouser leg. The third stopcock valve knob is located on the tube attached to the abdominal section. Normally, all three knobs will be in the closed (no airflow) position. Turn the stopcock valve knobs on all tubes to the open position (figure 7-9).

c. **Check Blood Pressure.** Check the casualty's blood pressure again before inflating the MAST.

d. **Inflate the Medical Anti-Shock Trousers.** If the MAST are used for the above indicated uses, all three compartments should be inflated until the Velcro closures begin to break away (a crackling sound should be heard). At this time, the patient should be monitored for response.

e. **Close Stopcock Valve Knobs.** Turn the stopcock valve knobs on the tubes to the closed position (figure 7-10). The pressure exerted by the MAST will remain equal and constant.

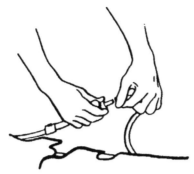

Figure 7-7. Connecting the air hose to a leg of the MAST.

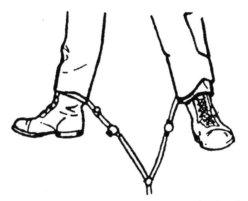

Figure 7-8. Trousers with both air hoses attached to the legs.

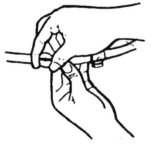

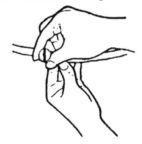

OPEN

Figure 7-9. Stopcock in the open position.

CLOSED

Figure 7-10. Stopcock in the closed position.

7-8. MONITOR A CASUALTY WEARING MEDICAL ANTI-SHOCK TROUSERS

a. **Initiate Intravenous Infusion.** An intravenous (IV) infusion should have already been initiated. If an IV has not been initiated, consider doing it now based on a good triage of medical supplies and your other patients.

b. **Monitor Vital Signs.** Continue to monitor the casualty's vital signs. The casualty's blood pressure should remain stable.

c. **Monitor the Medical Anti-Shock Trousers.** Look and feel for softness in the MAST. Listen for an active air release valve (loud, constant sound). If a section of the MAST looks and feels soft, inflate the section again.

d. **Deflating the Medical Anti-Shock Trousers**. Once the MAST has been applied to a casualty, it should not be removed unless a physician who is familiar with the MAST orders its removal.

Continue with Exercises

EXERCISES, LESSON 7

INSTRUCTIONS: Answer the following exercises by marking the lettered response that best answers the question or best completes the sentence or by writing the answer in the space provided.

After you have answered all of the exercises, turn to "Solutions to Exercises" at the end of the lesson and check your answers. For each exercise answered incorrectly, reread the lesson material referenced with the solution.

1. A soldier's skin is pale, wet, and cool. He is breathing at a rapid rate. He is very

   thirsty, but cannot drink because he feels as though he is going to "throw up."

   This soldier is probably suffering from _____.

2. When placing a casualty in a normal shock position, you should raise

   his_____ higher than the level of his heart.

   a. Feet.

   b. Head.

3. When treating a casualty for hypovolemic shock, you should loosen the

   casualty's clothing unless _____.

4. How should you position a casualty who has an open abdominal wound?

   a. Normal shock position.

   b. Knees flexed.

5. When inflating the MAST, you should inflate _____ sections at the same time.

6. You are inflating a MAST applied to a casualty. When should you stop inflating?

    a. The casualty's blood pressure stabilizes.

    b. You hear a loud, constant sound from the air release valve.

    c. The Velcro strips begin to crackle and stretch.

    d. Any of the above happen.

7. When should the MAST be deflated?

    a. Never.

    b. When the patient stabilizes.

    c. When ordered by a qualified physician who is familiar with the MAST.

8. A casualty has a severe head injury. What effect, if any, will this have upon your decision to apply medical anti-shock trousers to the casualty?

    a. No effect; apply the MAST.

    b. Apply the MAST, but inflate only to one-half normal pressure.

    c. The MAST should not be applied to the casualty unless ordered by the physician.

9. List six types of shock:

    _____   _____

    _____   _____

    _____   _____

Check Your Answers on Next Page

SOLUTIONS TO EXERCISES, LESSON 7

1. Shock (or hypovolemic shock).   (para 7-2)

2. a   (para 7-3e(2))

3. You are in a chemical environment.   (para 7-3f second Caution)

4. b   (para 7-3e Caution)

5. all three.   (para 7-7)

6. c   (paras 7-7 b, d, e)

7. c   (para 7-8d)

8. c   (para 7-5c(1))

9. Any six of the following

   Hypovolemic shock
   Metabolic shock
   Neurogenic shock
   Psychogenic shock
   Cardiogenic shock
   Septic shock
   Respiratory shock
   Anaphylactic shock.   (paras 7-1a, b(1) through (7))

End of Lesson 7

LESSON ASSIGNMENT

LESSON 8   Treating Soft Tissue Injuries.

TEXT ASSIGNMENT   Paragraphs 8-1 through 8-6.

LESSON OBJECTIVES   When you have completed this lesson, you should be able to:

    8-1.   Identify the primary functions of the skin and mucous membranes.

    8-2.   Identify common medical terms used to describe open and closed injures of the soft tissues and their meanings.

    8-3.   Identify procedures for treating open and closed soft tissue injuries.

    8-4.   Identify the procedures for stabilizing an impaled object.

SUGGESTION   Work the lesson exercises at the end of this lesson before beginning the next lesson. These exercises will help you accomplish the lesson objectives.

LESSON 8

TREATING SOFT TISSUE INJURIES

8-1. GENERAL

The term "soft tissue injury" is often used to describe an injury to the skin and/or mucous membranes.

a. **Skin.** The skin is the body's largest organ. The skin is watertight and bacteria cannot penetrate it unless there is a break (open wound) in the skin. The skin helps to regulate body temperature. The body is cooled in warm weather by the evaporation of perspiration and the dilation of blood vessels in the skin. In winter, the constriction of blood vessels in the skin helps to retain body heat. Specialized nerve endings transmit sensations such as heat, cold, pressure, pain, and position of the body in space. The three layers of the skin (epidermis, dermis, and subcutaneous layer) were described previously in paragraph 6-3a.

b. **Mucous Membranes.** Mucous membranes line all body openings (orifices) such as the nose, mouth, anus, and vagina. The mucous membranes perform the same basic function of protecting the body from invasion by bacteria that the skin performs. Mucous membranes secrete a watery substance called mucus that keeps the orifices lubricated.

8-2. IDENTIFY OPEN SOFT TISSUE INJURIES

If the skin or mucous membrane is penetrated, an open soft tissue injury exists. The injury can be an abrasion, laceration, avulsion, or puncture.

a. **Abrasion.** An abrasion is an injury caused by scraping the skin against a rough surface. The damage is usually confined to the epidermis and part of the dermis.

b. **Laceration.** A laceration is a cut or tear in the skin. The wound may extend through the subcutaneous tissue and into the muscle tissues. Major blood vessels and nerves may also be involved.

c. **Avulsion.** An avulsion is a tearing away of tissue. The separated part usually contains epidermis, dermis and subcutaneous tissue layers.

d. **Puncture.** A puncture is caused by an object such as a splinter, bullet, knife, or shrapnel penetrating the flesh. If the object goes through the body part and exits on the opposite side, the wound is called a perforated wound. If the object remains in the wound and protrudes above the skin, the object is said to be impaled. Even if the wound appears to be small and the bleeding does not appear to be severe, the object may still have caused significant internal damage.

e. **Amputation.** An amputation is the complete removal of tissue from the body. It may start as an avulsion type wound with a tearing away of the tissue, but once it is completely severed, the part is considered amputated. An amputation can also be complete separation of a limb from the body.

8-3. TREAT OPEN SOFT TISSUE INJURIES

Anytime the skin or mucous membranes are broken, the risk of infection is present. Also, open wounds usually result in more blood loss than do closed wounds. Treatments of major open wounds to the body have been discussed in previous lessons. Any open wound, however, can result in serious infection. The following are general procedures used in managing open injuries.

a. Keep the casualty calm and quiet.

b. Preserve any amputated parts.

(1) If the avulsed part is still attached to the body, replace the part in its bed (the wound from which it was torn) and cover the wound with a dressing. The avulsed part may still be receiving blood through the tissue remaining attached to the body.

(2) If the part is no longer attached to the body (amputated), retrieve the amputated part, wrap it in sterile gauze, and evacuate the part with the casualty to the medical treatment facility. If possible, keep the amputated part cool, but do not freeze the part.

c. Apply a dressing to control bleeding and prevent further contamination of the wound. If the wound is a puncture wound, look for both entry and exit wounds.

d. Stabilize any protruding objects (paragraph 8-4).

e. Immobilize the injured body part to reduce pain and further injury.

8-4. TREAT A WOUND WITH A PROTRUDING (IMPALED) OBJECT

If a foreign object is impaled in a wound, do not attempt to remove the object. Take measures to stabilize the object to prevent or reduce further injury and, at the same time, control bleeding. In some circumstances, it may be necessary to shorten the protruding object in order to move or evacuate the casualty.

NOTE: If an object is impaled in the casualty's cheek, the protruding object may be removed, but the casualty must be carefully monitored for bleeding into the mouth.

a. If the casualty is conscious, tell him to remain still and not move the impaled object.

b. Expose the impaled object by cutting or removing clothing to expose the wound site.

c. If the object is protruding from an extremity, check the pulse distal to the wound to determine if circulation is impaired. If circulation is impaired, evacuate the casualty as quickly as practical.

d. If there is serious bleeding from the wound, apply manual pressure to the wound to help control bleeding while you prepare to dress and stabilize the object. If possible, have a fellow soldier or the casualty himself apply the pressure while you dress the injury.

CAUTION: Do not exert force on the impaled object or on the tissue directly adjacent to the edge of the impaled object.

e. Apply a dressing to the wound using a field dressing or three sterile pads. The dressing helps to stabilize the impaled object and protect the wound.

(1) Field dressing. Use your scissors to cut a field dressing halfway through, slip the cut around the impaled object, and secure the field dressing with the attached tails.

(2) Three pads. Cut three sterile dressings halfway through. Place the first dressing around the impaled object (impaled object in slit as shown in figure 8-1). Place the second dressing around the impaled object, but coming from the opposite direction. Place the third dressing around the impaled object, but coming at a right angle to the first two dressings. If no additional bulky dressings are to be applied, secure the dressings with a roller bandage or cravat as described in paragraph g.

f. Apply additional bulky dressings, if needed to build up the area around the impaled object to further protect and stabilize the object. The bulky material may resemble a doughnut with the impaled object in the "doughnut hole."

g. Secure all dressings. Apply bandages, such as elastic bandages or cravats, to hold bulky dressings in place. The bandage should be tight, but not tight enough to interfere with blood circulation.

(1) If the wound is on an extremity, place a cravat under the limb with the center of the cravat on the side opposite that of the impaled object. Wrap the ends of the cravat around the injured extremity in opposite directions, covering the edges of the dressings. Tie the ends of the cravat away from the impaled object.

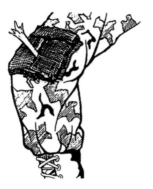

Figure 8-1. Applying dressings to stabilize an impaled object.

CAUTION: Do not anchor the bandage to the impaled object (that is, do not wrap the bandage around the object) or cause pressure on the object while applying the bandage.

(2)   If the wound is on a limb, recheck the casualty's circulation below the bandage. If circulation was not impaired before the bandage was applied but is now impaired, loosen and retie the bandage. Then recheck the circulation. If circulation is still impaired, evacuate the casualty as soon as possible.

h.   Immobilize the injured area. Apply a splint or sling if appropriate. Make sure the splint or sling does not cause additional movement of the impaled object.

i.   Take measures to prevent or control shock.

j.   Evacuate the casualty to a medical treatment facility.

8-5.   IDENTIFY CLOSED SOFT TISSUE INJURIES

In closed soft tissue injuries, the surface of the skin is not broken. Although soft tissue injuries can and do occur on any part of the body, they are common on extremities. Two common closed soft tissue injuries are contusions and hematomas.

a.   **Contusions.** Contusions (bruises) are usually caused by a blow from a blunt instrument (from a stick, for example) or by the body impacting with an object (falling to the ground, for example). The site of the injury normally turns "black and blue." The discoloration (ecchymosis) is caused by blood from the injury which is trapped and, with time, changes color. The site of the injury often swells due to the presence of blood and fluid leaking from the injured tissue cells (edema). Pain usually accompanies the injury.

b. **Hematomas.** A hematoma (blood tumor) is a localized collection of blood, often clotted, in the damaged tissues due to a break in the wall of a blood vessel. A hematoma is more serious than a contusion. Normal hematomas can contain more than 50 milliliters of blood and can often be palpated (felt with the fingers or hand). Severe hematomas, such as the internal bleeding associated with a fractured femur or pelvis, can contain a liter or more of blood and result in hypovolemic shock.

8-6. TREAT CLOSED SOFT TISSUE INJURIES

Minor bruises require no special care. If the injury is more severe, take measures to protect the injured area. If the injury is on an extremity, apply the following measures. The mnemonic device ICES (ice, compression, elevation, splint) may help you to remember the treatment procedures.

a. **Ice.** Apply cold (ice bag or chemical pack) to help reduce swelling and pain.

CAUTION: Do not apply ice directly to the skin. Applying ice directly to the skin could result in cold injury damage to the skin and underlying tissues. Use an ice bag or wrap the ice in cloth material to protect the casualty's skin.

b. **Compression.** Apply localized compression (elastic roller bandage or pneumatic counterpressure device) to help control bleeding and swelling. An elastic bandage can be applied to the injured limb using the techniques described in Lesson 2.

c. **Elevation.** Elevate the affected body part. If a fracture is involved, apply a splint before elevating the limb.

d. **Splint.** Apply a splint to the affected limb. If a fracture is involved, applying a splint is a must. Even if the limb does not have a fractured bone, applying a splint to the limb may help to reduce pain and prevent further injury. A pneumatic (air inflatable) splint can be applied to an extremity. The device will immobilize the suspected fracture and also apply pressure to help control internal bleeding.

Continue with Exercises

EXERCISES, LESSON 8

INSTRUCTIONS: Answer the following exercises by marking the lettered response that best answers the question or best completes the sentence or by writing the answer in the space provided.

　　　After you have answered all of the exercises, turn to "Solutions to Exercises" at the end of the lesson and check your answers. For each exercise answered incorrectly, reread the lesson material referenced with the solution.

1.　A casualty has a piece of wood impaled in his thigh. When dressing and bandaging the wound, you _____ wrap the bandages around the impaled object to help stabilize the object.

　　a.　Should.

　　b.　Should not.

2.　Unbroken skin and mucous membranes are the body's first line defense

　　against _____.

3.　Identify the medical term used to describe each of the following injuries to the skin.

　　a.　Skin is cut　　　　　　　　　　　_____

　　b.　Skin is completely torn away from the body　_____

　　c.　Skin is scraped　　　　　　　　　　_____

4.　A casualty has suffered large, soft tissue injuries to his leg and is in pain. There are no fractures present. Should you apply a splint to his leg before you evacuate the casualty on a litter?

　　a.　No, the splint will add unnecessary weight.

　　b.　Yes, immobilizing the leg will help to reduce pain.

5.　You are dressing a puncture wound on the casualty's leg. The wound has an impaled object. When should you check the circulation distal to the injury?

Check Your Answers on Next Page

SOLUTIONS TO EXERCISES, LESSON 8

1. b   (para 8-4g Caution)

2. Infection (or bacteria).   (para 8-1a, b)

3a. Laceration.   (para 8-2b)
  b. Amputation.   (para 8-2e)
  c. Abrasion.   (para 8-2a)

4. b   (paras 8-3e, 8-6d)

5. Before you dress the wound and after you tighten the bandages.
    (paras 8-4c, g(2))

End of Lesson 8